After the Cut

How to Prepare for and Recover
from Cosmetic Plastic Surgery

After the Cut™

How to Prepare for and Recover from Cosmetic Plastic Surgery

The Psomas Method™
by Nicole Psomas PT, MS, CLT/CDT

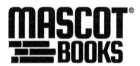

www.mascotbooks.com

*After the Cut: How to Prepare for and
Recover from Cosmetic Plastic Surgery*

Although the author and publisher have made every effort to
ensure that the information in this book was correct at press time,
the author and publisher do not assume and hereby disclaim any
liability to any party for any loss, damage, or disruption caused by
errors or omissions, whether such errors or omissions result from
negligence, accident, or any other cause.

This book is not intended as a substitute for the medical advice
of physicians. The reader should regularly consult a physician in
matters relating to his/her health and particularly with respect
to any symptoms that may require diagnosis or medical attention.

For more information, please contact:
Mascot Books
620 Herndon Parkway #320
Herndon, VA 20170
info@mascotbooks.com

CPSIA Code: PRFRE0219A
Library of Congress Control Number: 2018914695
ISBN-13: 978-1-64307-449-8

Printed in Canada

This book is dedicated to
Christopher Nicholas Tselepis

Table of Contents

Acknowledgments

To my father—who taught me the value of hard work, perseverance, and a good education.

To my mother—who taught me how to think outside the box and never take no for an answer.

To my brother—who always taught me to dream big and reach for the stars.

To my Yiayia Despina—who taught me no matter what I look like, I am beautiful and I am loved.

To my Yiayia Scillieri—who taught me to be thankful for the blessings I receive each day and to always wear lipstick.

To my family—who have been the columns that hold up the structure of my Parthenon.

To my friends—who have been an Oscar-worthy cast of characters in the movie of my life.

To Dr. David Shafer—without you none of this would be possible. You saw an opportunity to better your patient's recovery and quality of life and helped make all this possible.

To Graceanne Svendsen and Dr. Shafer's staff—thank you to the girl squad who supported me and always told patients exactly why they "must call Nicole."

To Georgia Giannopoulos—thank you for your mindful contribution using your vast knowledge of nutrition.

To Toni Gasparis and Elizabeth Resnick—thank you for your talents and editing contribution to this book.

To Ella Jordan and Danielle Morrone—my beautiful models who helped the book come alive.

To friend Larry Gutman—who has been the Goose to my Maverick, from Jefferson to NYP, to each of our professional endeavors.

To **Carolyn Padial, Delia Gorga, Lucia Boletti, Aida Osis**—who were not only my mentors but inspirational role models.

To **Mike Stype, Alex Bagley, Hope Hunter, Golda Widawski, Vickey Patel, Tracy Maltz, Danielle Gall, Robin Silver, Joe Russo, Ana Urso, Inna Tsykun, Stacey Coplan, and Lindsay Berman**—you not only built the foundation for my development as a therapist in different areas—you showed me how to push myself to be the best I can be.

To **Dr. Odell, Lisa Rivera, and Gina Sauro**—thank you for your dynamic leadership and dedication.

To **my physical therapy and occupational therapy colleagues**—for amazing support and teamwork—you have helped to develop my "can-do" spirit.

To **name a few doctors who inspired me professionally along the years**—Dr. Ulysses Scarpidis, Dr. Alyssa Golas, Dr. Kevin Smalls, Dr. Leslie Cohen, Dr. Jason Spector, Dr. Richard Swift, Dr. Dean Lorich, Dr. Peter Fabricant, Dr. Hanjo Kim, Dr. Philip Barie, Dr. Soumi Eachempati, Dr. Michael Marean, Dr. William Nugent, Dr. James Rosoff, Dr. James Wysock, Dr. Matthew Bott, Dr. Slava Gendel, Dr. Jared Knopman, Dr. Jeffrey Greenfield, Dr. Philip Stieg, Dr. Mark Souweidane, Dr, Michael Virk, Dr. Athos Patsalides, Dr. Caitlin Hoffman, Dr. Ilya Laufer, Dr. David Rubin, Dr. Jeffrey Perlman, Dr. Barry Kosofsky, Dr. Greg Dakin, Dr. Murray Engel, Dr. Anthony Watkins, Dr. David C. Lin, Dr. Jamie Green, Dr. Toni Beninato, Dr. Oriana Petruolo, Dr. Ashley Winter, and Dr. Nicholas Alexander.

To **the unsung heroes—the nurses**—you are the rock and foundation for patient care. You all inspire me and I am honored to call you my friends.

To **NYP**—which has taught me so much more than how to be a great therapist.

Thank you.

Foreword
A Message from the Team

A Note from
Dr. David Shafer, MD, FACS

A patient once asked me why I keep answering their questions with "we" instead of "I" when talking about their surgical plan. I explained that while I am the plastic surgeon, an entire team of professionals works together to maximize their surgical outcome. There are three phases to the patient experience: preoperative, operative, and postoperative. Each phase is essential in delivering a high level of patient care.

Neglecting to ensure smooth recovery during the postoperative phase can ruin the results of a flawlessly performed procedure. Considerable attention is placed on choosing the surgeon and the procedure and then, once the procedure is completed, patients are sent on their way and either lost to follow-up or left to fend for themselves. Figuring out how to care for themselves in their new condition is not only stressful and unproductive, but also is dangerous. Patients come up with home remedies, suggestions they have read on Internet message boards, or advice from family members who have no experience. Healing can be slower or results can be hindered by issues such as seroma—a pocket of fluid that develops in the body after surgery—which would otherwise be easily identified by members of the postoperative care team.

Early in my practice I was fortunate enough to cross paths with Nicole Psomas, who introduced me to postoperative physical therapy and lymphatic massage. As a double board-certified plastic surgeon performing surgeries ranging from facelift to liposuction to breast implants to mommy makeovers, a key aspect of my patients' recovery is the system put together by Nicole. Not only do the patients under her care return to their postoperative visits with less swelling, more energy, and more flexibility, but they also have a stronger awareness of their bodies and play an active role in their own healing process. In addition to the physical therapist-administered treatment, a key component is patient-administered treatment directed by Nicole. With proper instruction, patients can continue the techniques they have learned during their sessions, positively affecting their recovery process.

In this book, Nicole has compiled her years of experience working with postoperative patients. Her contribution to my patients' recovery process has been invaluable. Now, by reading this book, other doctors, physical therapists, and patients can use her special gift as a guide in the plastic surgery recovery process.

About Dr. Shafer

Dr. Shafer is a board certified in plastic surgery, a diplomate of the American Board of Plastic Surgery, and a member of the American Society of Plastic Surgeons.

Dr. David Shafer is trained in all aspects of plastic and reconstructive surgery. However, he specializes in cosmetic surgery.

Dr. Shafer has quickly made an impact in New York City and internationally. In 2009, he was featured in W *Magazine* as a

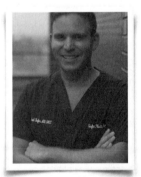

Photo 1: *David Shafer, MD, FACS*

beauty talent in plastic surgery and as one of the experts soon to be on your speed dial. Dr. Shafer developed the world's first plastic surgery-themed iPhone app. Dr. Shafer is a modern-generation surgeon and an innovator. He stays on the cutting edge of technological and surgical developments to offer his patients the best possible treatment and advice.

David Shafer's surgical training began at the Arizona Burn Center in Phoenix, Arizona. His research in wound healing and surgical techniques earned international attention and contributed to the scientific literature. Working with burn patients with complex wounds, Dr. Shafer focused on more than just survival. He concentrated on improving the patient's wellbeing both internally and externally. Improving a patient's appearance creates an enormous psychological boost. Many high-tech reconstructive developments in burn surgery, such as tissue engineering and tissue grafting, translate in a positive way to modern aesthetic surgery. As a graduating chief resident, Dr. Shafer was honored with all three possible awards including Intern of the Year, Rick Weimar Ambassador of Medical Ethics, and the Harry W. Hale Jr. Surgery Award for Outstanding Surgeon.

With a focus on plastic surgery, Dr. Shafer continued his training at the Mayo Clinic, which is consistently ranked as best in class for hospitals and surgical training. The international draw of this world-renowned medical center introduced Dr. Shafer to patients from the Middle East to South America to Asia. During this time, Dr. Shafer traveled to Hanoi, Vietnam to participate in the Global Health Organization's project to repair cleft lips and palates.

After the Mayo Clinic, Dr. Shafer was selected as an aesthetic surgery fellow at the Manhattan Ear, Eye, and Throat Hospital in New York City. This fellowship is recognized as one of the most prestigious fellowships in plastic surgery worldwide. Most plastic surgeons do not pursue specialized fellowship training. However, Dr. Shafer continued honing his surgical skills and knowledge rather than going directly into practice in order to achieve the best, most advanced training possible for cosmetic surgery. His traditional surgical training at the Mayo Clinic compliments the energy and innovation found in New York City.

The road from the Arizona Burn Center to the Mayo Clinic to the Manhattan Eye, Ear, and Throat Hospital has given Dr. Shafer a solid foundation in plastic surgery. In addition to teaching plastic surgery residents from New York University, Columbia University, Cornell University, and Lenox Hill Hospital, Dr. Shafer remains academically active. In recent years, Dr. Shafer has written peer-reviewed articles and chapters on facelift techniques, Botox Cosmetic®, Dysport™, and anesthesia for plastic surgery. Additionally, he has produced DVDs on Botox Cosmetic® injections to teach other surgeons fundamental skills and new developments.

A Note from Georgia Giannopoulos, RD, CDN, CNSC

When I first met Nicole several years ago, it was her bold personality that stood out. As I got to know her, I learned she was more than just an entertaining storyteller. In my experience working with her, Nicole is an individual passionate about her work, always striving to provide the highest level of physical therapy to those she cares for.

Often in life and especially in medicine, a team that works together toward a common goal is stronger than the sum of its individual parts. Along with others, Nicole and I have collaborated to provide specialized care to many individuals recovering from surgery. Nutrition and physical therapy go hand in hand—by optimizing both of these among other things, there is potential for phenomenal results.

Thank you for choosing to read this book and for taking us along on your journey. We hope you enjoy it.

About Georgia

Georgia is an award-winning registered dietitian based in New York. She holds a Bachelor of Science with distinction in research in nutritional sciences from Cornell University, and a Master of Science from New York University. Georgia is passionate about supporting individuals in meeting their personalized nutrition goals. To learn more, visit www.georgiagianno.com.

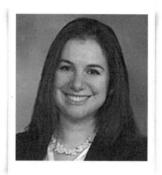

Photo 2: Georgia Giannopoulos, RD, CDN, CNSC

Introduction

For centuries, people have obsessed over maintaining youth and beauty. The search for the fountain of youth began in ancient times. Herodotus wrote about it. Philosophers, explorers, and the rich and powerful journeyed forth seeking it. Juan Ponce de León and Alexander the Great searched for it. Most recently, David Copperfield thinks he has found it. Today, in the fields of science and medicine, we have taken that journey into our own hands through plastic surgery.

According to the American Society of Plastic Surgeons, in 2017 approximately 1,790,832 plastic-surgery procedures were performed in the United States. This does not include minimally invasive procedures, i.e. Botox. An estimated total of 15.7 million cosmetic procedures are performed each year. This number has grown from the estimated 5.5 million total procedures performed in 2000. This shows that even though the American economy has declined in the past decade, the number of people getting plastic surgery has not.

Plastic surgery thrives on innovation. It continues to push ahead with new clinical breakthroughs, refinement of current techniques, and discovery of new ones. Plastic surgeons have recently begun to use lasers in certain surgical procedures. The use of lasers seems to have increased the number of people who choose to go under the knife. Lasers are called light scalpels and are used to perform procedures such as facelifts, skin resurfacing, and liposuction. Laser methods decrease bleeding and surgical scarring and reduce patient recovery time. Due to these medical advances, more people are likely to choose plastic surgery in the future. Those who previously felt the risks were too high may now feel more comfortable. More than ever before, a closer look at plastic surgery is in order, both because of the cost and because of what is involved in preparing for and recovering from it.

In 2009 I was an energetic, successful female living in New York City. I had a fulfilling life complete with friends, family, dating, and a job I loved. I took pride in my appearance. As a physical therapist, I understood the importance of staying healthy, working out on a regular basis, and maintaining a healthy diet. Even so, I felt like there were certain problem areas of my body that were not responding to diet and exercise. After researching it, I realized that genetics is a factor that can overpower any diet or workout routine. So I decided to think outside the box and explore a different route. I researched the best plastic surgeons in New York City. After careful consideration, I met with Dr. David Shafer of Shafer Plastic Surgery.

Right off the bat, Dr. Shafer and his team proved extremely professional and comforting. They provided me with good information. They explained how his services could be used to help me reach my goals. Due to genetics, I had a body shape where my waist and back were wider than my hips and buttocks. After my consultation with him, I decided laser liposuction was the best option. Laser liposuction would sculpt my abdomen and back to a shape more to my liking—a feminine hourglass shape. This was a better option—since I didn't have a large amount of fat to lose, this procedure had a shorter recovery time.

But I made the common mistake of assuming that a shorter recovery time meant no recovery time. I scheduled my surgery for the beginning of June, a week before my birthday. I wanted to look my absolute best for the party I planned, which included a hundred guests. I figured it was no big deal and I would be back on my feet in no time. I assumed it would be a quick outpatient procedure and that I would have some pain for a day or two, and then magically feel fine within a week. I thought it was kind of like getting your wisdom teeth out. I did not think there would be any work on my part, but I was wrong...

My surgery went perfectly and my doctor did a great job. Afterwards, my brother picked me up and brought me back to my apartment. Then I realized the reality of what recovery might require. The pain set in shortly after my anesthesia wore off. I needed to get the prescription medication filled from the pharmacy, but could barely move. I began to think, *Darn, why didn't I do this before surgery? What was I thinking? How am I going to go out and do this now?*

Oozing from my incision sites required changing my dressings regularly. I couldn't physically get myself out of bed, let alone change my own dressings or make myself something eat. When swelling set in, it became absolutely clear I could not do it alone. I had not prepared myself and needed my family to help me. Fortunately, I had family in my life that could drop everything, pick me up, and take me home to help me recover.

I have worked as a physical therapist at the top-rated New York-Presbyterian/Weill Cornell Medical Center since 2003. I have treated patients recovering from all types of surgery, including orthopedic surgery, heart surgery, and surgery after trauma. One group I often worked with were those recovering after reconstructive plastic surgery. I saw patients who had surgery just after cancer treatment, i.e. skin grafts, muscles flaps, and mastectomies. These patients had to follow a physical therapy protocol that might include learning to walk again, improving lung function, increasing range of motion, increasing strength, and decreasing swelling. The physical therapy treatments we provided helped patients to heal after surgery.

Lying on my couch, still swollen and draining, I felt I did not look how I expected. I was very swollen. I had pain and trouble moving. I was nervous about how I would make it to my birthday party in a week. An aha moment struck me—why was I looking at my surgery and recovery differently than the way I treat my patients after surgery? I realized that my skills as a physical therapist could be used to speed up my healing after cosmetic surgery. I could apply to myself the same advice I give patients after reconstructive plastic surgery. After realizing this, my recovery was a success. I could move better, I looked dramatically better, and I had less pain and swelling. I felt happy!

I did not expect the reaction I would get from Dr. Shafer at my one-week follow up visit. "Wow, you look fantastic!" he said. "You're so much further along than most patients immediately after surgery. You have less swelling and I can see the results of my surgery sooner."

"I used my techniques as a physical therapist to speed up my healing," I smiled.

His eyes grew wide and he beamed at me, "Can you do this with my other patients?"

I beamed back, "Sure. I'd love to."

He began referring patients to me. I performed treatments such as lymph drainage massage to improve swelling. I would also give education about what they could do for themselves. I would assign homework, including diet changes, exercises, and wearing the right garments. The feedback was great! Patients grew ecstatic! It was clear to both Dr. Shafer and myself that my input improved his patients' results.

But that wasn't good enough for me. As with most things in science and medicine, I wanted concrete evidence—objective data. So I began taking measurements. I would use a tape measure to assess the part of the body that had surgery. Then I would do my treatment session to reduce swelling. At the end of the session I would again measure the body part to see how many centimeters they had lost. This showed me that my treatment was working. I also took pictures before and after my treatment sessions to show what visual changes had occurred. Almost every single time after treatment, the patient would have smaller measurements and look better in pictures. This showed me that my treatments were not only making the patient feel better, but also making them less swollen.

As time went on, I realized most patients had no clue about the things they could do to speed up their recovery. I then wondered if others in the medical world knew of these treatments. This prompted me to take an advanced course on manual lymphatic drainage. I asked the instructor, "Do you think these techniques would help patients recovering from cosmetic plastic surgery?"

The instructor responded, "Well, I never thought of it—but yes, I'm sure it would be very beneficial to these patients."

I realized then that there was a major hole in a very popular area: recovery after cosmetic plastic surgery.

The field of physical therapy was born to help people recover after an injury.

When the human body is injured, it does not know whether the injury is coming from a mugger's knife or a surgeon's scalpel. The body only feels pain, and it responds by healing and repairing itself. Each injury goes through certain stages of inflammation and tissue healing. Physical therapists guide patients through each stage with different exercises and manual treatments. So why are physical therapists used after every type of surgery except cosmetic plastic surgery? They are regularly used after reconstructive plastic surgery. This is because cosmetic plastic surgery focuses on improving a person's appearance by choice and desire, and not out of necessity. This is wrong. Our mission as physical therapists is to make sure without judgment that patients have the right guidance, no matter what the reason they chose to have surgery.

This duty is reinforced by the guidelines of the American Physical Therapy Association, which state, "The physical therapy service has a statement of mission, purposes, and goals that reflects the needs and interests of the patients/clients served, the physical therapy personnel affiliated with the service, and the community...The physical therapy profession's commitment to society is to promote optimal health and functioning in individuals by pursuing excellence in practice." The American Physical Therapy Association attests to this commitment by adopting and promoting standards of practice for physical therapy. These standards are the profession's statement of conditions and performances that are essential for provision of high-quality professional service to society, and that provide a foundation for assessment of physical therapist practice.

Even though cosmetic surgery is used to change the appearance of a person, it is still surgery! It is important to understand the stages of healing because problems can occur if proper healing does not occur in each phase. Throughout this book, I provide guidance about what you can do to help proper healing during these stages.

This book has two purposes. The first is to inform you about how to prepare for plastic surgery, and the second is to teach you what you need to do after surgery to heal. The techniques I teach will help reduce swelling, help prevent complications, increase range of motion, and decrease lumps. They will help improve your results and appearance.

I have been fortunate to team up with a surgeon who understands the importance of proper postoperative care. Dr. Shafer also understands the benefits of properly educating the patient. In this book, I have used my years of experience to put together a guide that can be shared with surgeons, patients, and those considering plastic surgery.

If you decide that plastic surgery is the right choice for you, the steps discussed in this book will help you achieve the best results. You will be empowered to play the biggest role in your recovery!

Section One

Preparation Before Surgery

Chapter 1

What to Consider When Choosing Surgery

Is Surgery Right for You?

Why are you having plastic surgery? I can't answer that for you. Your significant other can't answer that for you. Your friends can't answer that for you. The decision to have plastic surgery is a personal one that only you can decide. It will have a significant impact on your life. It should be a serious decision.

Some people take months to decide on the right car or house. The decision to have plastic surgery should be made with the same level of consideration. It will permanently alter your physical appearance. This is not my opinion—it is a fact.

In order to make the right choice for yourself, there are questions you should answer prior to making any decisions. There are two types of plastic surgery: cosmetic plastic surgery and reconstructive plastic surgery.

Cosmetic surgery includes procedures to improve your appearance. Cosmetic surgery is usually elective surgery, chosen by the patient out of desire rather than necessity, i.e. breast implants solely for the purpose of increasing size. Reconstructive surgery restores form and/or function to any part of the body affected by birth defects, injury, or disease. An example of reconstructive surgery is breast augmentation and reconstruction after a double mastectomy for breast cancer. For the purpose of this book, I will be focusing only on elective cosmetic surgery.

Plastic surgery can create changes in your physical appearance as well as changes in self-esteem—hopefully positive, but that is not always the case. Generally, there are physical, emotional, and psychological factors that determine if a person is a good or poor candidate for surgery.

Who is a Good Candidate for Plastic Surgery?

From a psychological and emotional perspective, there are two categories of patients who are good candidates for surgery.

The first is a patient with a strong self-image and good self-esteem who is overall happy in their life. They may have a physical characteristic, typically one that stands out, that they would like to change. These patients usually feel good about themselves after surgery and maintain the positive self-image they had before.

Trish, a patient of mine, is a good example. Trish was a vibrant 24-year-old New Yorker. She had a successful job in finance, a solid group of friends, and was a physically active individual. She worked out four or five times a week, alternating cardio and Pilates. Overall she was very happy with herself, her lifestyle, and her place in life. The only thing that bothered her was the ring of fat around her midsection. She had tried for years to get rid of it through diet and exercise, but genetics overpowered her efforts. So after trying the conservative route, she chose liposuction of her midsection. She understood the choice she was making and the risk/benefits. After surgery she was extremely pleased with her results and continued to live a happy and productive life.

The second category includes patients who generally had positive self-image but, due to a cosmetic flaw, their self-esteem diminished over time. Surgery will allow these patients to slowly rebuild their self-confidence, though it may take some time. Although slow, a dramatic and positive change in self-confidence can result for these patients.

My patient, Jenny, is an example of this. Jenny was a pretty and outgoing girl. She was also very athletic growing up. She had a very non-descript nose until the age of 17 when she broke it playing soccer. A big bump developed on her nose, making her look very different. As time went on, people would say mean things to her about the size of her nose. She told me she would overhear people saying, "Oh you know Jenny—she's the soccer player with the big nose." This took a toll on Jenny's self-esteem. She did not want to be described by her nose. Over time she regressed from having an outgoing personality, to that of an introvert. After four years of living with the broken nose, she made the decision to have surgery. I worked with her after her rhinoplasty, and it was obvious her self-esteem did not change overnight. When I spoke with Jenny two years after her surgery, she was a different person. She said having her nose fixed was the best decision she ever made. She said it took time to rebuild her self-esteem, but now she feels like the person who she was meant to be. She is known for her vibrant personality, kind nature, and soccer talent—not for a big nose.

People in Good Health

People in good health are the best candidates for surgery. All surgery has risks but if you have a health problem, the possibility for a complication is greater. Healthy candidates for cosmetic surgery are:

1. Within 30 percent of their ideal weight
2. Non-smokers
3. Do not drink in excess
4. Emotionally stable, with low stress
5. Exercise regularly and maintain a healthy lifestyle
6. Patients who are active, strong, and in good cardiovascular health, i.e. have healthy hearts, will enjoy the best recovery from surgery.

Accepting the Disadvantages of Surgery

A good candidate also accepts the disadvantages of plastic surgery, which include:

1. Cost
2. Inconvenience
3. Pain and discomfort
4. Medical risk

Good candidates also have realistic expectations. They don't expect plastic surgery to drastically change their life. Recovery is much easier with a good support network.

If you do not meet all the criteria, it does not mean you won't be a good candidate for plastic surgery, but you may want to talk to your doctor about making some lifestyle changes before surgery.

Who is a Poor Candidate for Plastic Surgery?

Here is the reality: not everyone is a good candidate for plastic surgery, even though they may have a physical flaw that makes them appropriate for a procedure. One or more of the following things may make you a poor candidate.

Poor Health

Any and all health conditions should be discussed openly with your surgeon so they can help you make the most informed decision. It is important to let your doctor know your complete medical history. Some pre-existing conditions may make you a poor candidate for surgery.

People who have chronic health conditions—diabetes, hypertension, lung disease, heart disease, high cholesterol, severe arthritis, emphysema, and/or are malnourished, severely depressed, heavy drinkers, and/or smokers—are generally not good candidates for cosmetic surgery.

When discussing your medical history with your doctor you should also mention all of the following: medications; vitamins; hormones, i.e. oral contraceptives and estrogen replacement; herbal medications; alcohol; tobacco; and illicit drug use. These products can interfere with blood clotting or interact with medications used during surgery, and thus could cause major risks or death. You should also inform your doctor if you have a family history of strokes, blood clots, or clotting disorders.

Smokers

Smokers who choose to have surgery must quit for at least two weeks prior to surgery and remain smoke-free until at least two weeks after surgery for proper healing and recovery. Smokers have a higher rate of infection; skin separation (which is when the incision opens up rather than healing); skin death (which is also known as skin necrosis); and complications of anesthesia. One major study found that the risk of a significant area of skin death due to poor oxygen supply with a facelift in active smokers is increased by 1,500 *percent*—that's 1,500 times the risk for non-smokers.

Alcoholism

It is recommended that patients drink less than five ounces of alcohol a week. Alcohol thins the blood. Drinking alcohol before surgery could cause you to bleed-out during surgery and may cause death. Less serious risks include severe bruising. Consuming large amounts of alcohol after surgery can also cause serious side effects and really slow down the healing process.

Mentally or Emotionally Unstable

During a consultation, experienced plastic surgeons can usually identify those who are psychologically or emotionally unstable. A plastic surgeon may decline to operate on these individuals indefinitely or they may recommend the person get psychological counseling first. It is the responsibility of the surgeon to ensure that the patient's desire for a cosmetic change isn't part of an emotional problem that cannot be fixed by surgery.

Here are some examples provided by the American Society of Plastic Surgeons of patients who may be advised to seek counseling prior to surgery.

Patients in crisis

Those who have just gone through a traumatic experience such as divorce, the death of a loved one, or the loss of a job, are generally poor candidates. They may be looking to get results that cannot be achieved through a change in appearance. Attempting to overcome a crisis by changing your appearance is not a good solution. A patient must first work through the crisis and then determine a good reason for the desired physical change.

Patients who have a mental illness

Patients who show delusional or paranoid behavior may also be poor candidates for surgery, although surgery may be appropriate in these cases if it is determined that the patient's reasoning about surgery is not related to their psychosis. In these cases, a plastic surgeon may work closely with the patient's psychiatrist.

Patients with unrealistic expectations

This is the patient who walks in, saying, "I want Jennifer Aniston's nose" and expects to walk out of surgery looking exactly like her. Also, patients who want to look exactly like they did when they were a teenager. They need to understand that plastic surgery can help make the best version of themselves now. Hello—surgery is not a time machine.

Impossible-to-please patients

These patients consult with doctor after doctor, often seeking the answers they want to hear. They hope for a quick fix for a problem, which may not even be appropriate for plastic surgery—it might not even be a physical problem.

Patients who are obsessed with a very minor defect

These patients are born perfectionists. They may think that once that thing they hate is fixed, life will be fab! They may ultimately be an okay candidate for surgery, but first they have to accept the reality that it may never be exactly perfect. Also, these patients are at risk for becoming obsessed with plastic surgery and attempting to surgically fix every minor imperfection.

Patients who have Body Dysmorphic Disorder

Those with Body Dysmorphic Disorder (BDD) may not be the best candidates for plastic surgery. BDD is a body-image disorder characterized by constant obsession with an imagined or slight defect in one's appearance. It is a psychiatric illness affecting 2.4 percent of the population, and is more common than Bipolar Disorder or Schizophrenia. The American Psychiatric Association reports that as many as seven to 15 percent of patients undergoing plastic surgery have BDD. Persons with BDD who choose to undergo plastic surgery are generally not satisfied with the results, and often later become concerned about another body part.

Am I a Good or Bad Candidate for Plastic Surgery?

To get some idea about whether you are a good or bad candidate for plastic surgery, ask yourself:

Why do I want surgery?

What are my goals for surgery?

What do I expect plastic surgery to do for me?

Are my expectations realistic?

How will I handle unexpected results?

Do I feel fully informed about the risks and the specific considerations for the procedure?

Do I have the time in my schedule for proper recovery?

Can I afford the cost of plastic surgery?

Will the cost of the procedure add too much financial stress to my life?

Am I hiding my plans from friends and family? This can create added stress.

Am I having cosmetic surgery to please myself or someone else?

Is this something I have thought about seriously?

Have I explored alternatives to having surgery?

Do I have a support network to help me during recovery?

Am I willing to ask for help? Most people will need some help after surgery.

Understanding the Risks of Surgery

With any surgery there are general risks. This does not mean these complications will happen during your procedure, but it is important to realize that there are always risks. Plastic surgery is still surgery and should not be taken lightly. More specifically, there may be certain risks that come with plastic surgery.

Risks with Any Surgery

Complications of anesthesia/sedation

Some patients have serious reactions to the anesthesia or sedation used during surgery. Most anesthetic complications occur with general anesthesia. Patients who have heart trouble, lung disease, or are obese are at greater risk of complications due to anesthesia.

Airway obstruction

Anesthesia can sometimes irritate air passages, causing the vocal cords to spasm, which can block the airway. The anesthesiologist may need to insert a tube down the throat or cut into the windpipe.

Brain damage

Brain damage can occur if blood circulation is depressed to dangerous levels.

Malignant hyperthermia

This is a rare complication where body temperature, blood pressure, and heart rate all rise to high levels. If not recognized and treated quickly, it can lead to death. This is believed to be an inherited tendency.

Temporary paralysis

This occurs if muscle relaxants used as part of anesthesia have not fully worn off after surgery. It is easy to detect and easy to treat in the recovery room.

Aspiration

This occurs if you vomit during surgery and then the vomit is breathed or forced into the lungs. Aspiration can cause mild discomfort and can also lead to infections, chronic cough, lung obstruction, or pneumonia.

Blood loss

Bleeding is normal with any procedure. However, excessive bleeding can create major complications. If this occurs during surgery, your plastic surgeon and anesthesiologist will notice pooling blood and/or a blood pressure drop. If bleeding occurs after surgery, blood can accumulate under the skin and require an additional surgery. Talk with your doctor if you have any bleeding tendencies or clotting disorders, i.e. hemophilia.

Blood clots

A blood clot can be fatal. Longer operating time and general anesthesia increase the risk of a deep venous thrombosis (DVT), which is a blood clot in a vein. A DVT can occur as a result of a medical condition, or from immobilization, which allows blood to pool in big veins. Patients who have liposuction in their legs are at a higher risk. Although the specific risk is difficult to predict, the risk is greatly reduced by walking, doing ankle pumps, and changing position. Wearing compression garments also reduces the risk of a DVT.

Drop in blood pressure

Some decrease in blood pressure is normal during surgery. However, a sudden drop due to blood loss could lead to irregular heartbeat and possibly a heart attack.

Infection

The risk of infection is less than one percent, and antibiotics reduce this risk dramatically. However, if infection does occur, it is very serious. People who smoke, take steroids, or have certain vascular conditions are at greater risk. The longer your surgery lasts and the more blood you lose, the more likely you are to get an infection.

Loose stitches

If the stitches come loose, this can lead to internal bleeding. Such problems usually require additional surgery.

Other serious risks

Although these are very rare risks in healthy people, they can occur and you should be aware of them:

- Abnormal heart rhythm
- Heart attack
- Nerve damage
- Stroke
- Coma
- Death

Specific Risks with Cosmetic Surgery

All of the general risks of any surgery as described above, plus:

Skin death

Skin death, also called skin necrosis, usually follows an infection or a hematoma—a pool of blood under the skin. Skin necrosis is more likely among smokers. Skin necrosis is treated by removing the dead skin surgically, which may affect the cosmetic outcome.

Asymmetry

Moderate or severe asymmetries may require a second surgery. For example, one side of your stomach may have more fat taken out than the other side. Another example is if one breast is much larger than the other. Mild asymmetry is normal.

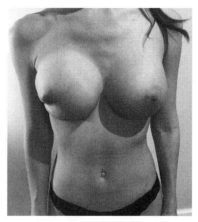

Photo 1: Breast asymmetry

Slow healing

Healing may be slower than expected due to age, genetics, diet, skin type, failure to follow doctor's advice, or factors beyond anyone's control.

Numbness and tingling

This often-temporary loss of or change in sensation is the result of injury to sensory nerves. Sometimes the loss may be permanent.

Irregularities, dimples, puckers, and divots

These can be due to surgical error, healing irregularities, or genetics.

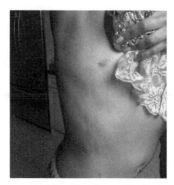

Photo 2: Irregularities, dimples, puckering, and divots

Seroma

A seroma is a pocket of fluid that collects under the skin. It can feel like having a waterbed under your skin. This most commonly occurs after liposuction or a tummy tuck.

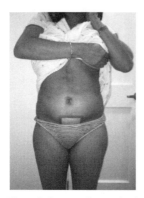 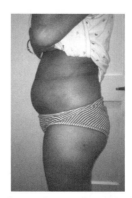

Photo 3: Seroma (example 1)   *Photo 4: Seroma (example 2)*

Understanding the Possible Psychological Effects of Cosmetic Surgery

Each of us has a self-image—a personal view of how we believe we look to others. People who are happy with their self-image are more likely to be self-confident, effective in work and social situations, and comfortable in their relationships. Research shows that those who have a poor self-image can tend to be less productive in their chosen activities, have greater inhibitions, and are overall more self-conscious.

Changing a small thing in your outer appearance can dramatically affect what happens on the inside. Plastic surgery can promote a stronger, more positive, self-image. The changes resulting from plastic surgery are often dramatic and permanent. Before your procedure is scheduled, it's important that you have a clear understanding of how surgery might make you feel and see yourself.

Postoperative Blues

Some patients may experience a low after surgery. This may range from mild feelings of unhappiness to more severe depression. Mild low feelings usually set in about three days after surgery. Some plastic surgeons call this condition "the third-day blues."

This low can be credited to a number of physical factors after an operation, including reactions to anesthesia and narcotic painkillers, pain and discomfort, or an undetermined biological process. Some other reasons are fatigue, stress, metabolic changes, and/or the frustration of waiting for visible and positive results. The low sometimes happens when you may be regaining your strength and endurance but you don't yet see the physical results you were hoping for.

Postoperative blues can last from a few days to a few weeks. Walking, light social interaction, and getting outdoors may help you get through this period faster.

Postoperative Depression

Postoperative depression is more severe. Patients who have a history of depression are more likely to experience this. Often they are already somewhat depressed before surgery, and the recovery from post-surgical depression is neither as guaranteed nor as straightforward as some surgeons expect. As a result, most people do not know that postoperative depression is a common complication of surgery.

Researchers have discovered that depressed patients are more likely to have other complications. They are less motivated to take an active role in their postoperative rehabilitation and recovery. No one knows exactly why there is such a strong link between surgery and depression. Some researchers think that many people experience post-surgical depression because it forces them to confront their own mortality.

Patients experiencing postoperative depression typically recover within six months of the operation, but during those six months, they may need medical or psychological treatment and they definitely need support. The treatment of postoperative depressive symptoms may vary but, no matter what the treatment, acknowledging the patient's feelings is crucial, and knowing what to expect in the postoperative period may help you cope better in the days following surgery, and thus lessen your risk for postoperative depression.

Reasons for Postoperative Blues or Depression

Emotional triggers of postoperative depression can be credited to disappointment in the outcome of the surgery, a negative response to physical changes such as stitches or scars, and resulting feelings of vulnerability and fear. Some examples of emotional triggers are:

- Guilt about the procedure
- Financial stress
- Rebound effect after the anticipation and stress of preparing for surgery
- Physiological effect of medications and anesthesia
- Physical trauma of the surgery affecting your emotional wellbeing
- Stress and fear about possible complications and changes in your appearance
- Feeling unlike your usual self because of postoperative restrictions on exercise
- The time it takes to adjust to your new look
- Dealing with reactions to your surgery from family and friends

Understanding the Realities of Plastic Surgery

Over the years I have heard the following thoughts and misconceptions about plastic surgery from patients, doctors, and friends as well as from my own experience. I have also included some statistics and facts so you can understand what is currently happening in plastic surgery.

Plastic Surgery is Real Surgery. Period.

Because it is real surgery, it requires weeks to months to heal—no matter what kind of surgery you have had. This is because after the body is cut, tissue healing begins. Tissue healing takes a minimum of four to six weeks in every single human body.

Remember that although the result from plastic surgery may be enhanced physical beauty, plastic surgery does not enhance inner beauty. True beauty begins inside oneself and cannot be shaped with a scalpel.

Having plastic surgery will not guarantee that you will attract a man or woman.

Having plastic surgery will not guarantee that you will keep that man or woman.

Plastic surgery will not automatically make you popular or liked, although it may give you more confidence, which could make it easier to make friends.

Some procedures may drastically change your appearance. It may take time for your mind to catch up with the physical changes in your body.

Some people believe that having plastic surgery was the best decision of their life—and some people believe having plastic surgery was the worst decision and biggest regret of their life.

To be certain if plastic surgery is the right choice for you, try all other options first—diet, exercise, detox, decreased drinking, and quit smoking. Really give it a solid effort. Don't go to the gym for three days or eat just a few meals from Jenny Craig and then claim it didn't work.

Plastic surgery can be very dangerous if not performed by a properly accredited and licensed surgeon.

Plastic surgery can be addictive.

Be prepared that people may not notice that you had work done. It might only be you, or a significant other, who is the most aware.

Be prepared that some people may notice and ask you if you had work done, even if you were not planning on telling people.

Be prepared that some people may express strong negative or positive opinions about plastic surgery.

Liposuction is a body-sculpting procedure. Having liposuction does not mean that you can't gain weight in the future. You can gain weight after liposuction, and weight gain may not go to the place where fat cells were removed—but it will go somewhere.

After liposuction, other parts of your body will get fuller and you will gain weight there first. It is hard to determine exactly where it will go. That is a gamble you take with liposuction.

Within months after my own abdomen sculpting procedure, my butt unexpectedly got fuller, like a lot fuller. This was a pleasant surprise— boys be like, "Damn!" So I just embraced my new Kim K. bod. But it's unavoidable that after liposuction the fat always goes somewhere else. For me, it worked in my favor.

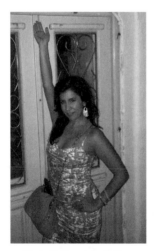 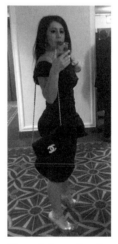

Photo 5: Buttocks before   Photo 6: Buttocks after
abdominal sculpting   abdominal sculpting

Understanding the Realities of the Recovery Process

General recovery

Recovery from any type of plastic surgery is not easy. It will take time and effort on your part. Those in their personal best physical shape, immediately prior to surgery, will have the best results and recovery.

The recovery can be gross. Bloody drainage oozes from incision holes that are held closed by stitches or staples. Some people go home with drains still in their body that will be removed days or weeks after surgery. The recovery can also be painful, so be prepared mentally for it. The first week after surgery is rough for every type of procedure.

You will see some positive results in about two weeks after surgery. You will see marked positive results in about six to eight weeks. You may not see maximum positive results for up to a year.

Heat and humidity will make you swell more. So, if you decide to have surgery in summer months, expect it to be more challenging.

Time off from work

You will need at least one week off of work—two is better. I always say two is better. For more invasive and involved surgery, some people may require more than two weeks. If you have a physical job, you will benefit from at least two weeks off work.

Garment wearing

If you aren't wearing your compression garment as often as recommended, you will not see maximum benefits. So many patients say to me, "I look fatter than before…that doctor messed up my liposuction." My reply is, "No, he didn't. You didn't wear your garment and now you have a lot of swelling and you're bloated. Wear your garment!"

Patients often mistake swelling for fat. Large amounts of fat are removed during a liposuction procedure, leaving an empty space. The body doesn't want an empty space so it naturally fills that space with fluid to maintain homeostasis. Wearing a garment compresses the body and decreases the fluid in that empty space. So when someone doesn't wear their garment, more swelling occurs. So—long story short—some people perceive this swelling as being fatter, but you are not bigger due to fat, you are bigger due to fluid swelling.

The garment can be very uncomfortable for some people. Some people have complained of feeling claustrophobic in the garment and have taken anti-anxiety medication prescribed for this purpose. It helps, did wonders for me since I am super claustrophobic.

Many people have said they can tolerate wearing the Stage 2 garment, i.e. Spanx®, better than the Stage 1 medical garment. It is very important to try and wear the Stage 1 garment for at least the minimum amount of recommended time, even if you feel it is uncomfortable.

Diet and fluid consumption

Water is your best friend—drink plenty of it!

Drinking alcohol before surgery will cause you to bruise a lot more. Alcohol thins the blood. This can also put you at risk for uncontrolled bleeding during and after surgery.

Some doctors say it is okay to drink alcohol after surgery, but remember alcohol has high sugar content and empty calories, suppresses the immune system, and causes bloating by making the body retain fluid.

Coffee, tea, and other caffeine-containing beverages are allowed but can dehydrate you if consumed in large quantities. Dehydration slows down healing. You want to be hydrated.

Your results will improve if you follow a low-sodium, high-protein diet, drink plenty of water, and consume little or no alcohol.

No smoking!

Smoking before and after surgery will be really bad for your healing, as will the use of tobacco or nicotine in any other form, even vapes! Put down the Juul! It takes longer to heal. The nicotine in tobacco, e-cigs, or vapes increases your risk for a blood clot and interferes with wound healing.

Pain medication can make you look bloated

One side effect of pain medication is constipation. This causes a patient to feel very uncomfortable and to look bloated. I always recommend that my patients wean off pain medication as quickly as possible, which should be done under the supervision of your doctor.

Exercise

You often must follow strict exercise guidelines. Strenuous exercise is not allowed for the first month.

Exercise should be carefully ramped up. Do not suddenly go from zero exercise to Crossfit. This will cause problems and complications.

Getting it on

Sex is often restricted for at least one week, and you may not feel up to it for a while.

If you feel ready for sex but wonder if it's allowed, always clear it with your doctor. Although you might not expect it, you may feel sore in certain body areas the day after sex.

Allowing yourself time to heal

Taking time to recover will improve your results. You will be more likely to have a good recovery if you get enough rest, follow garment-wearing schedules, walk after surgery, and eat a healthy diet.

After You Decide Surgery
is the Right Choice for You

Get Referrals

Finding the right doctor is essential for the best outcome.

Ask your primary doctor or other doctors you may know. Ask how many people they have referred to a particular surgeon and get feedback on the results.

Ask friends and family. Specifically try and find someone who has had the same procedure you are interested in having.

Contact a good hospital in your area and see who the surgeon on staff is. Hospitals will have a set of standards that will weed out unqualified doctors.

Check various websites. There are many websites that will rate doctors in your area and give you information about their training and specialties, and patients often will post testimonials.

Check the directory on the American Board of Medical Specialties (ABMS) website or call 1-866-ASK-ABMS (275-2267).

Choosing a Doctor

It is up to you to decide which surgeon is best for your specific goals, and selecting the right doctor is the best way to feel completely confident in the care you're going to receive. When choosing a plastic surgeon, consider the following factors:

Surgical experience

The surgeon:

- Should be board certified.
- Should adhere to a strict code of ethics.
- Must have at least five years of surgical training and experience, with a minimum of two years in plastic surgery.
- Should be trained and experienced in all plastic surgery procedures, including breast, body, face, and reconstruction.

- Should fulfill continuing medical education requirements, including updates on standards and innovations in patient safety.
- You also want to make sure a doctor does not have a history of malpractice.

Why Board Certified is Important

To ensure you are getting the proper care, you must choose a doctor who is board certified. In the US, doctors are typically certified by the American Board of Plastic Surgery. In Canada, they are certified by the Royal College of Physicians and Surgeons of Canada. All certifying boards require different amounts of surgical training and experience. All board-certified physicians are not trained equally for certain cosmetic surgery procedures. Some boards require extensive medical training and experience, such as the American Board of Plastic Surgery. Patients can be confident that physicians certified by either of these boards have specific and rigorous surgical education and training. Surgeons who have hospital privileges have already undergone the hospital's screening process and are required to be board certified.

Types of board certifications

The American Board of Medical Specialties (ABMS) is a not-for-profit organization that assists 24 approved medical specialty boards in the development and use of standards in the ongoing evaluation and certification of physicians. ABMS is recognized as the "gold standard" in physician certification and believes higher standards for physicians means better care for patients.

The American Board of Plastic Surgery (ABPS) is overseen by the ABMS. The ABPS certifies physicians in plastic surgery of the entire body, including the face, neck, and full body. These physicians must undergo the strictest surgical training requirements and have the highest standards of certification for plastic surgery procedures for the whole body and face, including procedures such as breast implants, tummy tucks, and facelift surgery.

The American Board of Facial Plastic and Reconstructive Surgery (ABFPRS) certifies physicians in the field of facial plastic and reconstructive surgery. These board requirements for certification are specifically related to surgery of the face, head, and neck, especially procedures such as facelift and rhinoplasty.

The American Board of Otolaryngology (ABO) certifies physicians in the specialty of otolaryngology (ear, nose, and throat, or ENT) as well as head and neck surgery.

Designations the Doctor May Have

In order to become a physician, each student must complete four years of undergraduate training, four years of medical or osteopathic school, and additional years of internship and residency. Many MDs and DOs receive graduate medical education in a particular specialty through a paid residency that they complete in a hospital. Many DOs participate in a 12-month internship and a residency that may be extended to a total of six years. To be licensed in the United States, physicians must graduate from an accredited medical school, pass an examination, and receive one to seven years of graduate education, depending upon their specialty. In order to receive board certification by the American Board of Medical Specialties (ABMS) or American Osteopathic Association (AOA), the physician must pass another examination within two years of practice.

Doctor of Medicine (MD) degree

A doctor of medicine has completed a four-year course of study at a medical school, learning traditional medical theory and practice. In traditional medical practice, diseases and health are evaluated and treated based primarily on symptoms or signs specifically associated with a health condition.

Doctor of Osteopathic Medicine (DO) degree

A doctor of osteopathy has completed a four-year course of study at an osteopathic school, learning holistic medicine as well as traditional medicine. Osteopathy is a non-invasive, drug-free, hands-on medicine that focuses on total body health as well as treatment and strengthening of the musculoskeletal framework. This includes the joints, muscles, and spine.

Fellow of the American College of Surgeons (FACS)

This means that the doctor's education, training, competence, and ethical conduct have passed an intensive assessment consistent with the standards of the College of Surgeons. The doctor may also have completed more training in a sub-specialty.

The Surgical Facility Where the Doctor Operates

It is recommended that the procedure be performed at an accredited medical facility. An accredited facility is one that must meet strict national standards for equipment, operating room safety, personnel, and surgeon credentials. Plastic surgery performed by board-certified plastic surgeons in accredited facilities has an excellent safety record.

Importance of accreditation

Accredited ambulatory facilities have:

- An extremely low rate of serious complications (less than one percent)
- An extremely low mortality rate (less than one in 57,000)
- The advantage of lower costs
- Around-the-clock care by a minimum of two or more licensed staff members at all times
- A defined emergency plan is defined ready to be implemented
- Necessary equipment and medication on site to handle any complications
- Staff members who are certified in Advanced Cardiac Life Support (ACLS)

Questions to Ask at the Initial Consultation

Coming to the initial consultation prepared with the right questions will use the doctor's time and your time efficiently. Many doctors will charge an initial consultation fee of approximately $100 to $300 on average. If you are not prepared, it may be your money that is also wasted. Remember, an informed patient can make informed decisions. Don't feel shy to ask questions. It is your right to ask your doctor questions—you are not burdening them.

When I first thought about my decision to consider plastic surgery, I felt overwhelmed. I did the necessary research online but I still had a lot of questions and felt nervous I wouldn't remember them when I went for my consultation. I remember the best piece of advice I got was from one of the doctors I work with. She said, "Nicole, every time a question pops in your head, write it down. This way by the time you go in for your consultation, you will feel like you had all your questions answered." I did that and she was right. I felt very calm and informed after my first meeting with the surgeon.

Questions about the Doctor

How long have you been practicing?

How many procedures do you perform a year on average?

Where did you go to medical school?

Where did you study plastic surgery as a specialty and for how long?

Are you board certified?

Are you certified by the American Board of Plastic Surgery (ABPS)?

What facilities do you operate in? Are you affiliated with any major hospitals or medical centers?

What do you do to continue your education and training in plastic surgery?

What are your standards of ethics and practice?

What is your area of expertise?

Questions about the Procedure

Am I a good candidate for this procedure?

What is the cost?

What are the risks?

Can I see before and after photos that are similar to the surgery I desire?

Do you use computer imaging to personalize the look I wish to achieve?

What usually happens during the surgery?

How long does the procedure take?

What type of anesthesia is used?

Will there be an anesthesiologist?

Where will the incisions be made?

Where will the procedure take place? In an office or a hospital?

Questions about Recovery

How much pain can I expect?

What is the recovery time?

How much time will I need off from work?

How long until I see results?

How long will the results last?

How will this affect how I look in clothes or how clothes fit?

What are my options if I am dissatisfied with the results?

How are complications handled?

Ask about Follow-Up Care

Every doctor should see patients for follow up after their surgery. This is so they can properly examine the results, and determine if you are healing well and progressing properly without infection. Most commonly a doctor will request to see a patient within one week of the surgery date. The number and frequency of additional visits will be determined by the doctor. This is based on the extent of the surgery, any postoperative concerns, and the rate of your recovery.

Ask about the Cost of the Surgery

Understand with plastic surgery there is always going to be a fee. The fee may vary from surgeon to surgeon. Some doctors may offer a payment plan. Some may require you to pay half in one payment and the balance in a second payment. Question if the quoted price is negotiable. It may or may not be.

The temptation is to go for the doctor who has the cheapest price. When having plastic surgery, getting the cheapest price may not be the wisest choice. Plastic surgery is often permanent or hard to reverse. It is an alteration to your face or body. You could look like this forever! Therefore, higher quality is more important than the best deal. Surgery can often be pricey, so many surgeons will offer financing or a payment plan. A payment plan is better than a sale. This is the only time in life I will say that—and it's true! It is important to ask the doctor if any of the fees can be covered by insurance.

Please, please hear me on this topic! I am a girl who loves a sale. I once got a pair of Jimmy Choos during Black Friday for $100—for real. I love a bargain! But when it comes to plastic surgery, never ever go for the cheapest price! I cannot stress this enough. I have seen the results on people who went cheap on their plastic surgery. They went for the discount—they went to the Dominican Republic or they used an assistant instead of the plastic surgeon—and it showed! Most patients I know who went the discount route ended up having to pay double to get their surgery reversed.

Okay, I'm going to confess—one time only I tried lip injections. There was a medical person in training (I won't say who) living in my building. He offered to do the injections for $100 if I would recommend him to my friends. Well let me tell you, it was a nightmare. Afterwards I had to pay $1,500 to a top Park Avenue plastic surgeon to get it reversed. Thank goodness it could be reversed.

So leave the sales for Black Friday. Pay market price when it comes to plastic surgery.

National average surgeon fees in 2017 (American Society of Plastic Surgeons)

Breast augmentation...$3,718

Breast implant removal $2,357

Breast lift (maxoplexy)..$4,672

Breast reduction $5,482

Buttock implants..$4,884

Buttock lift..$5,113

Calf augmentation $3,707

Cheek implant...$2,837

Chin augmentation $2,236

Dermabrasion..$1,170

Ear surgery (otoplasty)..$2,909

Eyelid surgery (blepharoplasty)..............................$3,026

Facelift (rhytidectomy)..$7,448

Forehead lift..$3,374

Hair transplantation (2013 statistic).......................$5,136

Lip augmentation (non-injection)............................$1,665

Liposuction ....$3,374 (per area)

Lower body lift..$7,679

Nose reshaping (rhinoplasty) $5,125

Pectoral implants $4,196

Thigh lift...$4,857

Tummy tuck (abdominoplasty) $5,992

Upper arm lift...$4,223

Chapter 2
Preparing Your Body, Mind, and Home Before Surgery

Now that you've made the decision that plastic surgery is right for you and you have chosen a surgeon and scheduled surgery, it's time to prepare yourself. Even though you know that surgery is the best option, it is natural to have fears and questions about the process. In this chapter I discuss the pre-operative (before surgery) steps required to prepare you physically, emotionally and psychologically.

Knowing that there are ways for you to prepare for surgery will empower you—you have the power to facilitate your healing and recovery. And what is the best way for you to heal? Proper preparation!

Preparing Your Body

After scheduling your surgery date, the doctor will recommend pre-surgical or pre-admission testing. This means that a physical exam will be performed and your overall health will be examined. A series of tests will be needed.

It is important to let your doctor and healthcare provider know if you have had blood tests, urine analysis, or an EKG (electrocardiogram) in the last 30 days. If you have, this may eliminate the need for more tests to be done. If you have the results of any of these tests in your possession, you should send them to your doctor or take them with you to the pre-surgical visit.

Pre-Surgical Physical

Tests performed at the pre-surgery physical may include:

- Medical, alcohol, tobacco, drug, and medication histories
- Physical exam of heart, lungs, and airway
- Blood work
- Urine analysis (to check for infections)
- EKG (heart test)
- Chest X-ray, depending on your age
- Update on flu shot or other vaccinations
- Review of a written physical provided by your primary medical provider, saying you are cleared for anesthesia and surgery.

A friend of mine was prepared and scheduled for male breast reduction surgery. After his pre-admission blood work was done, the doctor noticed he had irregularities on his EKG. He never knew he had a heart issue until this came up. The surgery had to be cancelled because he was too high risk to go under anesthesia.

There are important facts the doctor must know prior to you having surgery. This could change how the doctor performs the surgery, determine if you are allowed to have surgery, or trigger a bad side effect from surgery if your doctor does not know about a specific fact.

Examples of questions the doctor may ask you at the physical

What prescription medications are you taking? Are you taking any non-prescription medications? Medications you are taking in your day-to-day life could interfere with surgery or cause a bad reaction. Let your doctor know about any prescription medications or non-prescription supplements that you are currently taking.

Do you have any allergies to drug or food groups? If yes, what are you allergic to?

Are you allergic to latex? Latex is a substance found in many hospital and surgical materials, i.e. surgical gloves.

Have you ever had surgery before? Did you have complications from that procedure?

Have you had anesthesia before? If so, were you allergic to any anesthetic drug? Do you know if any blood-relative has had problems with anesthesia?

Do you have any pre-existing conditions such as heart, lung, or kidney problems; strokes; or liver damage?

Have you had any previous blood transfusions, diabetes, high blood pressure, jaundice, or depression or other psychiatric disorders? It is also important to tell your doctor whether you have sleep apnea and use a breathing machine while sleeping. Also tell your doctor if you have any loose teeth or dental work, such as bridges or crowns.

How much and how often do you use alcohol? Tobacco or nicotine? Illicit drugs? All of these can make a big difference in the safety of anesthesia and surgery, plus affect your recovery negatively—so be honest with your doctor about your use.

Know What to Put in Your Body

Good food

Maintaining a well-balanced diet is essential to prepare for any type of surgery. Providing your body with the proper nutrients helps strengthen your immune system, which will result in a faster recovery.

When preparing for surgery, get to your ideal weight! The better shape you are in before surgery, the better the results after surgery.

Eat a diet high in protein, vitamins, and other nutrients—this speeds up healing.

Don't eat foods high in sodium right before surgery, i.e. Chinese food or sushi with soy sauce. High-sodium foods will make you bloat a lot more right after surgery.

If your surgery is bariatric, i.e. gastric bypass surgery, a more specific diet is indicated. For optimal healing, candidates for abdominoplasty, more popularly known as tummy tuck surgery, should be as close to their ideal weight as possible before surgery.

Stop smoking and any other use of tobacco or nicotine

You should stop smoking two weeks before anesthesia and surgery. Smoking affects your cardiovascular system in two ways that concern anesthesiologists—oxygen carrying capacity and infection. It increases the amount of carbon monoxide attached to hemoglobin in the blood, which displaces oxygen that would otherwise be attached to the hemoglobin. Hemoglobin carries oxygen throughout your body. If that oxygen supply is decreased, your heart may slow down dangerously. Smoking also increases your risk for infection.

Nicotine increases the amount of oxygen that your body needs. But your oxygen supply under anesthesia decreases so your body's extra need for, but lack of, oxygen will threaten your wellbeing under the knife. On the topic of oxygen, smoking can make the lungs more prone to collapsing during surgery.

The good news—studies show that once you stop smoking, your body recovers from smoking within 12 to 24 hours. Carbon monoxide in the body significantly decreases and most of the nicotine that is in the bloodstream is eliminated. So you will decrease your risk for complications significantly if you stop smoking at least two weeks before your surgery date!

No alcohol or caffeine

I know that you need your morning cup of coffee and your glass of wine at night may seem like a necessity, but these can affect you badly when it comes to surgery. Caffeine can raise blood pressure and alcohol is a blood thinner, so cutting back on both is a good idea before surgery.

It is recommended not to consume an alcoholic beverage for at least 72 hours before surgery. I recommend patients stop drinking one week before surgery. Alcohol should not be consumed right after surgery because this may trigger post-operative bleeding.

One of my patients went on vacation to Puerto Rico the week before her liposuction surgery. Like many people on vacation she drank margaritas, beer, and mixed drinks. She said she wanted to have fun before surgery. She is lucky this was not a deadly mistake. She also did not tell her surgeon she drank that much right before surgery. She could have bled out during surgery—luckily she didn't—but she did suffer bad side effects. Her legs were so swollen and bruised that she looked like she was run over by a car. I said to her, "Why would you drink alcohol right before surgery? Would you drink like this if you were getting your appendix out?" She replied, "I just didn't think of liposuction on my thighs as real surgery."

It goes without saying that you should be clean and sober from all illicit drugs for at least two weeks, and preferably longer, before anesthesia and surgery.

Vitamins

In addition to all of the other recommendations above, doctors recommend something else—taking a multivitamin. A multivitamin can supplement your body with vitamins, minerals, and other nutritional elements it will need more of than usual during the stress of surgery and healing.

However, some vitamins can harm you if taken right before surgery, even if they are normally good for your body. On page 50, I will inform you of the vitamins that can be harmful.

Medication

It is important to make your doctor aware of all medications you are taking prior to surgery because they could cause bad side effects during surgery. If you are currently on a medication—prescribed or over the counter or even a non-prescription health supplement—ask your doctor if you should keep taking it before or after the operation.

Certain medications should not be taken before an operation. Anything containing aspirin or ibuprofen is not allowed before or after surgery because it can cause an increase in bleeding.

Acetaminophen, i.e. Tylenol, is commonly allowed. Your doctor will usually prescribe a pain medication that contains acetaminophen unless you have an allergy to it.

Coumadin is another blood-thinning agent. If you are on a Coumadin regimen, it is very important to discuss this with your doctor.

Some steroid sprays, i.e. Flonase or Nasonex, may impact surgery as well.

Antibiotics are commonly prescribed to prevent infection post-surgery.

For certain surgical procedures that do not require anesthesia, your doctor may prescribe a light sedative that you will have to take on the day of surgery. It is a good idea to get all your prescriptions filled prior to your surgery day—you don't want to deal with going to the pharmacy while you are in pain.

Homeopathic and naturally occurring medications may also interfere with your surgery and with some medications that are routinely used during plastic surgery. Because most homeopathic agents are not approved by the US Food and Drug Administration (FDA), this is a controversial subject. So, before taking any such medications, please discuss them with your doctor.

Two common homeopathic medications that are used in plastic surgery are Arnica and Bromelain.

Arnica

Arnica montana is a mountain flower that grows around the world. It is used as a naturopathic remedy that not only helps prevent bruising but also aids in clearing bruising that has occurred after surgery. Arnica has been used for over 100 years, both as a topical ointment and as an oral supplement. Applied externally, it reduces bruising and muscle soreness. When taken by mouth, it helps reduce and clear bruising as well as speed healing after surgery. In the past decade Arnica has received increased attention as some recent research has shown its benefits. Healing properties have been credited to many of its over 100 components. Arnica contains chemicals, called sesquiterpenes, which have anti-in-

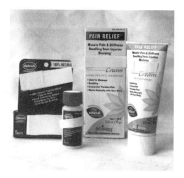

Photo 1: Arnica Montana

flammatory benefits. Arnica also contains antioxidant flavonoids, carotenoids, and silicic acid, all of which are all believed to have healing properties. It can routinely be taken pre- and post-surgery. However, always consult with your doctor before taking any medication.

Bromelain

Bromelain is a homeopathic anti-inflammatory containing the proteolytic enzyme found in pineapples. Proteolytic enzymes are capable of dissolving proteins. Bromelain is most often used to help reduce swelling *after* plastic surgery

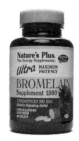

Photo 2: Bromelain

Do not take Bromelain *before* surgery as it can increase your risk for bleeding. Take Bromelain after any plastic surgery procedure to help reduce swelling. However, always consult with your doctor before taking any medication.

Medications to Stop Before and After Surgery

All of the medications you are currently taking should be specifically cleared by your doctor. Any medication listed below should be discontinued 14 days prior to surgery. Do not stop it on your own. Stop it under guidance of your doctor!

If you use herbal medications and supplements, you still need to clear them with your doctor. Studies have found that less than 10 percent of all users of herbal supplements inform their doctors before surgery. Often, people believe that since herbal medications and supplements are promoted as natural, they are safer and less likely to cause side effects than prescription medications. This is not always the case. Many herbal medications and supplements can significantly increase bleeding during and after surgery. This not only adds to the length of the procedure, but also increases the risk of infection, postoperative pain, and scar formation. So—and I cannot stress this enough—please tell your doctor about anything and everything you are putting into your body!

Avoid Vitamin E

It is important that you not take any vitamin E for about two weeks prior to surgery because it can cause bleeding. Normally, vitamin E helps decrease the risk of heart disease; but in the context of surgery it can lead to increased bleeding. Wheat germ, nuts, and some vegetable oils contain the largest amounts of vitamin E—so look out for it on food labels!

It is recommended that all homeopathic, herbal medications and herbal teas be discontinued prior to surgery. Here are just a few that can cause complications:

Medication	Can Cause the Following During Surgery
Ephedra/ Ma huang	Seizures, heart attack, stroke; interfere with anesthesia
St. John's wort	Heart failure; interfere with anesthesia

Kava	Coma; interfere with anesthesia
Ginkgo biloba	Bleeding in brain and spinal cord
Licorice	Heart attack, increased bleeding
Garlic	Increased bleeding
Ginger	Increased bleeding and increased blood sugar
Ginseng	Increased bleeding and decreased blood sugar
Omega-3, EFA, flax, and fish oil	Increased bleeding
Vitamin E	Increased bleeding; decreased wound healing
Glucosamine and Chondroitin	Increased bleeding
Dong quai	Increased bleeding
Saw palmetto	Increased bleeding
Feverfew	Increased bleeding
Bromelain (*if taken before surgery*)	Increased bleeding
Valerian	Delirium; heart failure; prolonged sedation
Goldenseal	Prolongs sedation; sun sensitivity
Echinacea	Prolongs sedation; poor wound healing

Get Your Garment

Get your garment ahead of time. Before surgery you will need to be fitted for and purchase a compression garment. This can be done at a local surgical supply store. Items necessary for dressing changes can also be purchased there, including non-stick pads, gauze, antibacterial soap, and non-adhesive tape. I will discuss garment wearing in detail in future chapters.

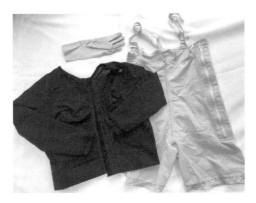

Photo 3: Examples of garments

Preparing Your Mind

As the human body has evolved over the years, we have developed certain responses to protect ourselves from changes in the environment. In today's times we do not face the same pressures for survival as our ancestors did, like being killed by dinosaurs or dying of smallpox, which triggered our body's natural defense mechanisms. We do encounter threats and fears in today's society in different ways, like taking a test, getting mugged, or having surgery.

Whether today or hundreds of years ago, our unconscious response to protect ourselves is controlled by our autonomic nervous system. It is made up of both the sympathetic and parasympathetic nervous systems. What exactly are these nervous systems? What do they do? How do they do it? Why are they important to you and your surgery?

How the Autonomic Nervous System Works

The autonomic nervous system (ANS) affects heart rate, digestion, urination, salivation, perspiration, diameter of the pupils, and sexual arousal. The ANS is made up of the sympathetic nervous system (SNS) and the parasympathetic nervous system (PNS). The SNS's general action is to induce the fight-or-flight response. This response to stress mobilizes the body and puts it into action. So, for example, if a mugger comes at you, your body immediately starts to produce extra adrenaline. This increases the delivery of oxygen and glucose to the heart and large skeletal muscles, so you can fight or run away. Your heart beats faster and harder, and your airways widen to make breathing easier. Your body releases stored energy in the form of glucose and your muscle strength is increased. Your palms sweat, your pupils dilate, and your hair stands on end. At the same time, body processes that are less important in emergencies, such as digestion and urination, are slowed. Your immune system goes into overdrive because with the need for fight or flight comes increased risk of injury and possible infection.

The PNS balances the SNS by increasing the activity of systems that cause us to "rest and digest" and "feed and breed." The PNS controls body process during ordinary situations. The PNS is responsible for sexual arousal, salivation, lacrimation (tears), urination, digestion, and defecation. It generally conserves our energy and restores our body. At rest, your heart rate slows and your blood pressure decreases. Your digestive tract processes food and eliminates wastes. Energy from the processed food is used to restore and build tissues.

How Stress Going into Surgery Affects You

Whether you are stressing about work, a relationship, or surgery, stress is never a good thing. Psychological stress negatively impacts your body. It can have an adverse effect on your health by weakening your immune system because of the triggering of the SNS.

Many events that happen to you and around you put stress on your body, and you can put stress on yourself.

Stress can be triggered by your environment, (work, school, etc.), your body (weight gain/loss, your image, etc.), and your thoughts. Studies have shown stress can heighten the risk for upper respiratory infection, worsen autoimmune disorders, cause headaches, elevate blood pressure, cause heart problems, trigger skin conditions, cause depression, and trigger anxiety. All of these health problems can have a bad effect on your impending surgery, so it is important to relax.

How Anxiety Going into Surgery Affects You

You've decided to have your surgery, you've thoroughly prepared, and—even after all that prep work—you're still anxious. This is common, and you are not alone. But you need to try to reduce anxiety before surgery because it can badly affect you during and after surgery.

Research studies have found that more anxiety before surgery means more pain after surgery. Studies show that pain after surgery was dramatically lower in patients that were more relaxed going into surgery. So do yourself and your body a favor: relax in order to reduce your pain.

A study of patients having knee replacement surgery found that anxiety not only causes more pain but also poorer recovery in getting knee function back. Even though this study was done on knee patients, and not cosmetic surgery patients, it shows that the recovery is worse for patients who are anxious going into surgery.

Anxiety before surgery was also the factor that increased pain from two to 30 days after breast surgery. Other studies found that after elective Caesarean deliveries, preoperative anxiety negatively affected the mother's speed of recovery and satisfaction. Stress and anxiety can do several things to your body that will badly impact you during surgery. They will put your body's systems into fight-or-flight mode. This can cause problems during surgery, such as increased heart rate, increased blood pressure, increased breathing rate, and increased blood sugar.

How Depression Going into Surgery Affects You

Studies have shown that depression and neuroticism were factors that caused increased pain after surgery. Neuroticism is the tendency to be in a negative emotional state for a long period of time. People with neuroticism tend to have more depressed moods. They also are known to frequently suffer from feelings of guilt, envy, anger, and anxiety more often and more severely than other people. Neuroticism is commonly referred to as "being neurotic."

Importance of Preparing Your Mind

You cannot control most of the actions of your ANS because they are involuntary and spontaneous, such as breathing, but some of the responses of the ANS work together with the conscious mind. For example, if you are having thoughts about something scary, this can cause your heart to race. If you think calming, peaceful thoughts, perhaps about the time you were sitting on the beach in Miami, your body will relax and your heart rate will slow down. Preparing yourself psychologically prior to surgery can train your body to remain calm.

This means that if your body relaxes, it will not trigger all those negative effects. This can produce positive outcomes, such as better wound healing, less need for pain medications, less time in the hospital, fewer surgical complications, and an overall better surgical outcome.

Consider the following interventions to reduce your response to stress and anxiety:

- *Relaxation training*: Meditation is an example of relaxation training.
- *Guided imagery*: Self-directed thoughts and images can guide and focus your mind into a relaxed state.

- *Empowerment and self-efficacy*: You can train your mind to believe that you will succeed at the goal you set. In this case, the goal is successful surgery.
- *Education*: Preparing your mind by getting information about what to expect from surgery and during recovery will help put you at ease.

Preparing Your Home Environment

Having a prepared home before surgery will help you after surgery. You want your house to be accessible and ready before you arrive home after surgery. You may feel lethargic or nauseated, and have pain or soreness and lifting restrictions, so you will need to have everything waiting for you at home. You also cannot drive after surgery—so this means no trips to the store because you forgot to fill a prescription, get a post-op garment or simply pick up milk. You will need someone—a friend or family member—to pick you up from the hospital or doctor's office to assist you home. You are not allowed to drive a car or operate machinery for at least 24 to 72 hours after surgery, so prepare for this.

I definitely recommend that you have someone at home to help you for the first few days.

When I first came home from surgery, I didn't have anyone to help me. I didn't think I would need it—but then I panicked when I couldn't get out of bed myself. I could barely get to the kitchen—forget cooking! Luckily my family lived over the bridge in New Jersey. I called them and they were able to drop everything to help me. What if I didn't have that? I would have been stuck! Don't put yourself in a position to get stuck!

The number of days you need assistance will depend on the extent of your surgery. Some people hire a nurse or aide to care for them for the first few days after surgery. If this sounds like an appealing option, set it up in advance. Your doctor may have a nurse or other personnel to recommend.

Prepare food

You will be in pain and unable to move easily, so food will be the last thing on your mind, but when your stomach starts rumbling, you will want to be pre-prepared! You can prepare meals ahead of time so they are easily accessible and ready to go, or you can have food delivered.

Be mindful about what you order as take-out. Food prepared in restaurants may be filled with empty calories and high sodium content—exactly what you don't want in your body! Another option is meals prepared for you by a generous friend or loved one.

Tip!

Cook meals ahead of time and freeze them in individual containers. This way you can pull out one meal, defrost it, heat it, and then eat! This is a healthier option than take-out.

One client told me she thought she was doing a good thing by stocking her freezer full of those pre-packaged diet meals, to eat after surgery. Big mistake—those pre-packaged diet meals are usually super-high in sodium. This patient was so bloated after surgery and she couldn't figure out why. When I pointed out her poor food choices, she immediately stopped eating those meals—and her swelling got better.

Prepare a resting space

You will be spending a lot of time resting, so preparing that space is a good idea. If you have a surgical procedure that does not allow you to lie flat, you should have enough pillows to prop yourself up in a semi-reclined position. Consider purchasing a wedge or bed-rest pillow so you can prop yourself up more comfortably.

Once you are in a comfortable position, consider entertainment—your magazines, books, iPod, laptop, and television remote should all be within reach! If someone is there to help you, consider using a bell or intercom to signal your need for assistance.

If you have your bedroom or living room on a different floor than your bathroom, you may want to consider staying on one level. It may be difficult to frequently go up and down stairs.

You may require assistance to get in and out of bed, to get to the bathroom, or to take a shower. If walking to the bathroom is too difficult, you may want to purchase a bedside commode (portable toilet).

Prepare medications and supplies

Get all prescriptions filled ahead of time—those that you will need to take before and after surgery.

Some medications will need to be taken the morning of surgery. One example is an anti-nausea medication that is taken the morning of your surgery.

Get a supply of surgical cleansing soap and sponges that you will use to wash your body with the morning or night before surgery.

Keep the pre- and post-op instructions that your doctor gives you in a handy place.

Get a supply of Arnica and Bromelain ahead of time—for before and after surgery. Remember:

1. Arnica tablets are taken before and after surgery.
2. Arnica cream/gel is used after surgery.
3. Bromelain is taken after surgery only, not before surgery.

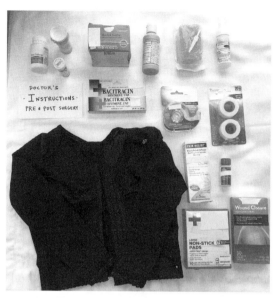

Photo 4: Organize all supplies and instructions before surgery (see above).

Prepare ice

I highly recommend that you prepare ice for your recovery at home. Gel packs or thick plastic bags filled with crushed ice can be used. You may want to have multiple ice packs to cover the entire affected area all at once. When one bag of ice melts, it is wise to have more ice already prepared and ready to use. Double up freezer bags to prevent leaking.

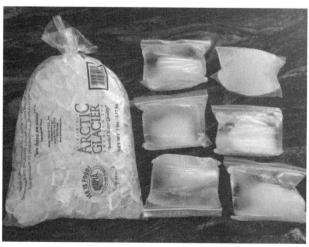

Photo 5: It's important to prepare your supply of ice before you need it (see above).

Tip!

For facial surgery, such as rhinoplasty, a bag of frozen peas works well because it easily conforms to the curves of your face.

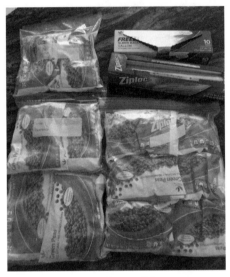

Photo 6: Use packages of frozen peas to ice facial surgery sites (see above).

After all this body, mind, and environment preparation, you will be ready to tackle your surgery day with ease!

Chapter 3
Diet and Nutrition

I am not a nutritionist, not a registered dietician, nor an official expert in this area. But over the years as a physical therapist, I have educated my patients about the role diet and nutrition play in the recovery process after injury or surgery. I have given my patients tips on modifying their diet to get the best results while rehabilitating. I have found a very specific diet plays a major role in the results after cosmetic plastic surgery. I place my patients on a strict high-protein/low-sodium diet which allows them to see maximum results ASAP.

When I got involved in plastic surgery recovery, I had no idea just how important the food choices post-surgery were until I experienced it myself and saw the effect it had on patients. I cannot stress this enough—it is so important!

This chapter will teach you about how your diet will affect your healing. If you follow the recommendations that the dietician and I make in this chapter, you will see the best you after surgery!

Recommendations by a Physical Therapist

Recommendation #1: Eat Low Sodium

Soup is your enemy! If I could make only one point about

recovery after any plastic surgery, it would be this: eat low sodium. By the way, sodium is salt. Eating a low sodium diet is the secret to looking good after any plastic surgery. I promise you, you will thank me. It is as simple as this—eat low sodium! Change your mindset this very minute. Forget the Atkins diet. Forget Jenny Craig. Forget it all. Of course, you must eat healthy and I will go into that, but this is the most important thing you need to do after cosmetic surgery—eat low sodium!

I have known many patients resistant to this change. They were eating tons of soup and sushi, insisting it was low in calories and fat. But then they would cry to me each session, saying, "Nicole, I look worse than I did before surgery. I am so huge." I would tell them, "No, you aren't fatter—you are swollen! Stop eating salty foods!" Finally, they would switch their diet to low sodium—and then I would get the phone call: "Oh my God! You were right!! I look amazing!"

Read the labels on the foods you eat. Check the Nutrition Facts guide. Some of the lowest calorie foods have the highest sodium content.

You can find Texas A&M University's guide "The Sodium Content of Your Food" online. I refer all my patients to this chart. It lists common foods and their sodium content. What you find there will shock you.

Try to follow a diet that is consistent with a "cardiac" or heart-healthy diet. The recommended amount of sodium is less than 1500 mg a day.

Warning! Be careful if you normally have low blood pressure. Check to make sure your blood pressure does not drop too low if you are eating a low-sodium diet. Some signs of low blood pressure: dizziness; lightheadedness; fainting; poor concentration; blurred vision; nausea; cold, clammy, pale skin; rapid, shallow breathing; fatigue; depression; thirst.

The 10 highest-sodium foods

Stay away from these!

Salts

Table salt

Baking soda

Baking powder

Sauces and salad dressings

Soy sauce

Reduced-salt soy sauce—
it's not very reduced!

Fish sauce

Teriyaki

Oyster sauce

Hot pepper sauce

Steak sauce

Reduced-fat salad dressing

Barbeque sauce

Worcestershire sauce

Hamburger relish

Salted butter

Just stay away from most
sauces and dressings except
oil and vinegar

Cured meat and fish

All cured meats

Bacon and turkey bacon

Dried beef

Salami and Italian salami

Prosciutto

Beef jerky

Salt cod

Salted mackerel

Canned anchovy

Smoked salmon

Smoked whitefish

Caviar

Smoked herring

Sushi of any kind—just do
yourself a favor and walk
on past the restaurant.

Cheese—regular and processed

Roquefort and blue cheese

Queso seco

Romano and Parmesan

Feta

Camembert

Gouda

Cottage cheese

American

You name it!

Pickles

Any type of pickle—sweet, dill, kosher, etc.

Olives

Pickled eggplant and other pickled vegetables

Jalapeno peppers

Sauerkraut

Regular and instant soups

Soup is your enemy unless it's homemade and low sodium!

All canned soups

Instant soup crystals and powders

All bouillons

Roasted and salted nuts and seeds

Salted peanuts

Almonds

Cashew nuts

Sunflower seeds

Pistachio nuts

Pretzels and chips

Most pretzels—read the label!

Potato chips

Doritos®, etc.

Sesame sticks

Reduced fat chips

Salted popcorn

Soy chips

Pita chips

Fast food and pizza

Any kind of fast food. You will be shocked at the amount of sodium in fast food. For example, McDonald's® Bacon Clubhouse Chicken Sandwich has 1,720 mg of sodium. The Big Breakfast with Biscuit has 2,150 mg of sodium— that's insane!

Canned vegetables

Any canned vegetable unless the label says "Low Sodium" or "No Salt Added." Even then, check the actual sodium amount.

Beverages

Gatorade® and other sports drinks

Sodas and fruit-flavored drinks

Cocoa mix, hot chocolate, and flavored coffees

Low-sodium food options

Choose these low-salt food items after surgery.

Breads, cereals, rice, and pasta (without sauce)

Whole grain bread

Granola—read the label carefully.

Puffed rice

Rolled oats

Shredded wheat

Unsalted popcorn

English muffins

Breadsticks without salted tops

Fresh fruit that is particularly low in sodium

Apples

Bananas

Blackberries

Cherries

Peaches

Pears

Raspberries

Watermelons

Fresh vegetables—any fresh vegetable, these are the lowest in sodium

Broccoli

Cabbage

Cauliflower

Chickpeas

Cucumber

Green peppers

Lima beans

Sweet potatoes

Protein

Six ounces daily of any fresh or frozen beef, veal, lamb, pork, poultry, or fish, prepared without salt or skin

Low-sodium, water-packed tuna or salmon

Eggs and egg substitutes

Unsalted nuts and seeds

Low-sodium nut butter

Fats

Olive oil and other cooking oils	*Unsalted butter or margarine*
Low-sodium mayonnaise	*Low-sodium salad dressings*

Dairy

Milk contains virtually no sodium. Choose fat-free or low-fat milk and yogurt more often than cheese, which can be high in sodium. Milk and yogurt are also good sources of potassium, which can help lower blood pressure.

Low-sodium cottage cheese	*Cream*
Fat-free or low-fat yogurt	*Non-dairy creamers*
Skim or one-percent milk	*Sour cream*
Soy-based drinks with added calcium	*Ice cream*

Condiments and extras

Choose condiments that are low in sodium or have no sodium at all.

Try seasonings instead of salt to flavor food.	*Low-sodium chili sauces*
Vinegar	*Mrs. Dash and other sodium-free seasonings*
Lemon	*Yeast*
Fresh horseradish or horseradish prepared without salt	*Jams and jellies*
Cream of tartar	*Low-sodium ketchup*
Mustard	*Low-sodium tomato sauce*
Tabasco sauce	*Vegetable juices without salt or sodium added*

Spices

Bay leaf	Onions
Curry powders	Paprika
Dry mustard	Parsley
Garlic	Pepper
Ginger	Rosemary
Herbs, such as basil, mint, chives, or tarragon	Sugar (use very small amounts)

Tip!

Some of your favorite snacks may come in an "Unsalted" version.

Recommendation #2: Eat Protein

This is the other recommendation I make to patients: protein, protein, protein! To put it simply—eating lean protein helps you heal better, but when choosing high-protein foods, remember to make sure they are also low in sodium!

Foods high in protein

Lean turkey and chicken	Tofu
Fish	Beans
Low-sodium cheese	Yogurt, milk, and soymilk
Lean beef and veal	Nuts and seeds

Recommendation #3: Stay Hydrated

Drinking plenty of water after surgery has many positive effects. The human body is sixty percent water. So we need water to function at our best.

Immediately after surgery, drinking water helps flush the

anesthesia out of your body. In the days after surgery it helps flush out swelling.

I tell my patients to forget soda and forget juices—drink water!

You also have to be careful that some of the beverages you are choosing aren't working against you by dehydrating your body. Large amounts of coffee, tea, or other caffeinated beverages can dehydrate you. Alcohol dehydrates you.

One of my patients, Chloe, was a 22-year-old model who had liposuction on her stomach and back. Her first appointment with me was one week after her surgery (I usually meet with patients sooner). When she arrived for her first appointment with me, she showed up crying. She began by saying she made a big mistake having surgery and that she is now fatter than she was before surgery.

I began by taking her history. I asked her to describe her normal diet to me. She replied, "I am an extremely healthy eater...I only eat organic...I'm into juicing...I'm a vegetarian. I also try and eat food low in calories." I said, "That's great, but give me examples of the foods you have been eating after surgery." She replied, "I have been eating tons of vegetable soup and sushi. They're low-fat and I figured these are good foods when you are not feeling well. I also have been drinking a lot of tea and coffee." Right then I knew what her problem was—her diet. Before I examined her body, I knew she was not fat—she was just very swollen. The foods she had chosen were extremely high in sodium, which causes swelling. She also was not flushing her body with water. Coffee and tea are very high in caffeine, and when consumed in large quantities can dehydrate your body.

I then examined her stomach and back—exactly as I suspected. She was extremely swollen. Her skin was stretched and tight with a blanched (whitish) appearance. It was also hot when I touched it. These are signs of excessive swelling. I told her, "Chloe, you have to change your diet. You have to cut out the soup and sushi—and start drinking more water." She agreed to more water, but was really against not eating soup and sushi. She insisted that this is what she always eats and it's low in fat and calories. I told her she had to change her mindset right now—it's more important to focus on low-salt foods. She finally agreed.

One week later I got a phone call from Chloe: "Nicole, you were right. I lost five pounds in four days. I did what you said, and I just kept peeing and peeing. I feel and look amazing!"

Recommendations from a Registered Dietician

Eating well before and after surgery is vital for optimal healing. Choosing to eat nutritiously can help you look and feel great. Now is a great time to assess the health quality of the food choices you make.

Do you enjoy a variety of foods to get nutritional benefits from them? Are there any nutrients you're not getting enough of? Are you prepared to eat nutritiously after surgery to support your body as it heals?

I will review some of the basics of nutrition as it relates to preparing for and healing after cosmetic surgery. Please note the information provided is general and not intended to replace the advice of your physician and registered dietician (RD).

The best way to get the variety of vitamins and minerals your body needs is through food. Before surgery, work with your physician and registered dietitian to assess if you are deficient in any vitamins or minerals and if you can resolve this by eating more of certain foods or supplements.

As you are planning for surgery, speak with your physician about any vitamin, mineral, or herbal supplements you may be taking. Most of the time, these need to be stopped at least ten days (check to make sure) before surgery as they may interfere with anesthesia. Always check with your physician first before resuming supplementation after surgery, as supplements may interfere with other aspects of your treatment plan.

Q: Is a registered dietitian (RD) the same thing as a nutritionist?

A: Registered dietitians may refer to themselves as nutritionists, but not all nutritionists are registered dietitians. An RD is a nutrition expert credentialed by the Academy of Nutrition and Dietetics; to earn this credential, one needs to complete required dietetics coursework, an accredited dietetic internship, pass an exam, and then participate in continuing education to maintain certification. To find an RD, ask your healthcare team for a referral or visit www.eatright.org.

Keeping a food diary may be a helpful way to keep track of what and how much you are eating and how you feel, both physically and emotionally, when you consume different foods and beverages. Some prefer to physically write a food diary with a pen on a piece of paper or journal, others prefer to use an app (i.e. My Fitness Pal).

Starting with the Basics

Water

Water is a vital nutrient and one that is often overlooked.

How much fluid do you need every day? This varies from person to person based on many factors, including age, sex, physical activity, climate, and medical history.

Looking at the color of your urine is a good way to assess if you are drinking enough fluid or not; when the urine is dark yellow/very concentrated, that's a sign that you need to consume more fluid.

If you are feeling thirsty, you're already dehydrated. As people age, their perception of thirst decreases, so an older person may not feel thirsty but may actually be dehydrated. Some people, such as those with kidney disease or congestive heart failure, may need to limit the amount of fluid they consume. If you're not sure of what your fluid goal should be, speak with your registered dietitian.

Water is one of the preferred fluids because it's naturally zero calories and refreshing. To add some flavor to your water, try infusing it with fresh fruit and/or squeezing some lemon into it. Many fruits and vegetables are packed with water; these also help keep you hydrated.

Water content of some popular fruits and vegetables

Here are some popular fruits and vegetables and their water content:

Watermelon	92%
Cucumber	96%
Strawberries	92%
Zucchini	95%
Grapefruit	91%
Celery	95%
Cantaloupe	90%
Radish	95%
Peaches	88%
Tomato	94%
Raspberries	87%
Sweet peppers	92%
Pineapple	87%
Eggplant	92%
Apricots	86%
Cauliflower	92%
Blueberries	85%
Broccoli	91%
Plums	85%
Carrots	87%

Getting your groceries

You may not feel like food shopping after your procedure. To make eating nutritiously as simple as possible, set yourself up for success and go grocery shopping in advance. Stock your kitchen with nutritious foods that you can eat postoperatively; by having the foods on hand, you will be a lot more likely to eat them. Think of simple recipes that will not require a lot of prep;

for example, something like a shake made with Greek yogurt and frozen fruit—easy, nutritious, and delicious.

If you prefer to order take-out, study menus for local delivery or take-out places ahead of time, so you know what is available to you, and identify choices that are nutritious. If you're not sure about how a dish is prepared (often it is not specified on menu), just ask!

The most important thing, whether you are ordering take out or making food at home, is to have everything prepped and ready before surgery.

Salty facts about sodium

Fluid retention or swelling is a common complaint for many people after plastic surgery. Moving around/getting exercise and reducing the amount of sodium you eat can help you reduce fluid retention. The Dietary Guidelines for Americans recommends limiting sodium intake to 2,300 milligrams (mg) per day. Some people, including those with high blood pressure (hypertension), may need to further limit the amount of sodium to 1,500 mg per day.

When you eat too much sodium, your body may hold onto extra fluid. This may feel uncomfortable and it may make it harder for you to participate in your physical therapy sessions or otherwise move around. Eating too much salt can cause your body to hold onto excess fluid, which can make you look puffy and make you feel weighed down.

Salt is an acquired taste. Your taste buds turn over every 10 to 14 days. So, although lower sodium foods may initially taste bland if you are used to eating higher sodium foods, your taste buds will renew themselves and after a few days a food you may have enjoyed in the past may taste too salty to you.

Prepare yourself going into the procedure by gradually decreasing the amount of sodium you eat, if you eat too much. A study found less than ten percent of the salt we eat comes from that which we add with the salt shaker at the table; most of the salt we eat comes from processed foods or foods prepared outside of the home. That being said, it's still a good idea to taste food before adding extra salt to minimize extra sodium you may not even need for flavor.

The foods that tend to be highest in sodium are those that are salted, smoked, brined, or pickled, plus packaged foods including canned and boxed items, as salt is often added to preserve the food and increase the shelf life.

Some packaged foods that do not taste salty are actually high in sodium, such as bread. You can find the amount of sodium in milligrams on the Nutrition Facts label of packaged foods, so this is a good place to check if you are monitoring how much sodium you are eating.

Sodium-filled soup

Often when patients are not feeling well after surgery, they go to a common healing food—soup. But soup after surgery is your enemy! Soup will make you bloated and retain fluid. Soups are commonly loaded with sodium, depending on the brand and how it is prepared. One cup of soup may have roughly 800 mg of sodium—or more. If you love soup and sodium is something you need to limit, do not fret. There are plenty of lower-sodium soup options out there. You just have to find ones that you enjoy. Doing this before surgery can make it a lot easier after surgery.

Canned foods can secretly add sodium

Many fresh foods, such as fruits, vegetables, beans, and legumes, are naturally low in sodium. Choosing frozen fruit and vegetables (without added flavorings) instead of canned is a way to help avoid added salt. When using canned foods, look for no-added-salt options and/or rinse them with water to reduce the salt content before adding them to the recipe or eating them.

Skip the salt—add flavor without sodium

If you like to cook, a great way to add flavor to dishes without added salt is via herbs, spices, and citrus flavors, like lemon or lime. Some popular herbs are oregano, parsley, mint, and rosemary. Oregano is a common ingredient in Mediterranean cuisine and goes well in salad. Parsley is a great way to season soups and vegetables. Mint tastes very refreshing—especially when blended into drinks and smoothies. Rosemary is versatile and pairs well with chicken and fish among other ingredients. Onions and garlic are also packed with flavor.

Condiments containing sodium

Some condiments are also packed with sodium. For example, soy sauce contains a whopping 1,000 mg sodium per one tablespoon—that's approximately half of the sodium most people need for the entire day! Ketchup has roughly 150 mg per tablespoon and mustard roughly 170 mg per tablespoon. You don't need to avoid these items—you just need to be mindful of the amount you use if you are trying to limit your sodium intake.

Salad dressing contains roughly 250 to 350 mg sodium per two-tablespoon serving. For less sodium and fewer additives, try something like extra-virgin olive oil and red-wine vinegar instead, which provides minimal sodium. Add oregano, cucumbers, tomatoes, and onion—and you have yourself a gourmet Greek salad (without the cheese)! Olives are delicious and provide heart-healthy fat, but may contain anywhere from 20 to 100 mg sodium per olive depending on the size and type, so consider limiting them if you are looking to limit your sodium intake.

Other secretly hidden sodium

Another source of hidden salt is foods that do not necessarily taste salty. For example, a plain New York-style bagel gives roughly 500 to 700 mg of sodium, depending on its size and the ingredients used—add an ounce of cream cheese and that's another 120 mg of sodium. A slice of bread contains roughly 150 mg of sodium—if you use two slices to make a sandwich, there's 300 mg sodium without any of the fillings.

True or false: Kosher or sea salt has less sodium than table salt.

False! Kosher or sea salt has roughly the same amount of sodium as table salt. The difference is that kosher or sea salt comes in larger granules, so some people say you may use less in a recipe.

Vitamins C is Key

Vitamin C is essential for collagen formation and wound healing. Studies have shown that without adequate vitamin C, wounds will not heal.

The recommended dietary allowances (RDAs) for vitamin C in adults are 90 mg for a male and 75 mg for a female. Some people may require more vitamin C, up to 2,000 mg/day, if they are healing wounds, thus forming a lot of collagen. Some people, including those with hemochromatosis, glucose-6-phosphate dehydrogenase deficiency, and renal disorders, may need to limit their vitamin C intake. If you have one of these illnesses, you should check with your doctor about proper Vitamin C intake.

Some foods that provide the highest amount of vitamin C are guava, yellow and red peppers, kiwi, oranges, strawberries, and papayas. Even kale provides a fair amount of vitamin C, approximately 87 mg of vitamin C per cup.

Amount of Vitamin C in some popular vegetables

Here are some examples of the amount (in mg) of Vitamin C in some vegetables:

Guava..376.7 per cup

Yellow pepper ....341.3 per large pepper

Red pepper.............................190.3 per cup chopped pepper

Kiwifruit....................................166.9 per cup sliced kiwifruit

Navel orange ....97.5 per cup orange sections

Strawberries ....89.4 per cup strawberry halves

Papayas ....88.3 per cup of 1" pieces

Scotch kale, raw........................87.1 per cup of chopped kale

Don't Forget about Vitamin A and Zinc

Research suggests having inadequate amounts of vitamin A and zinc may also impair wound healing.

Vitamin A is found in sweet potatoes, carrots, pumpkin, butternut squash, collard greens, and kale, among other foods.

Zinc is found in oysters, beef, wheat germ, sesame seeds, lentils, soybeans, and pine nuts, among other foods.

Your physician and registered dietitian can help evaluate if you are eating enough of these nutrients and if you have a predisposition for developing deficiencies for any reason.

Before starting any vitamins, minerals, or herbal supplements, speak with your healthcare team to ensure there are no contraindications. Some over-the-counter supplements may make you feel sick, interfere with healing, and cause even more dangerous side effects.

More Diet Dos and Don'ts

If you feel bloated after surgery, you may want to avoid using drinking straws, drinking carbonated beverages, eating foods containing sugar alcohols, and/or eating fibrous foods such as beans and some vegetables because they will make you bloat even more.

Constipation Cures

Some people develop constipation after surgery. In addition to physically moving around, something that may help alleviate this is consuming enough fluids and dietary fiber. Fiber is generally found in the skins and seeds of raw fruits and vegetables, nuts, seeds, and whole grains. The daily goal for dietary fiber intake for many adults is roughly 25-35 grams.

Some fibrous foods and grams (g) of dietary fiber per serving

Beans (i.e. navy, yellow, kidney, French) ...... 23-25 per ½ cup

Chickpeas .... 17 g per ½ cup

Barley .... 8 g per ¼ cup (dry)

Bulgur .... 6 g per ¼ cup (dry)

Quinoa .... 3 g per ¼ cup (dry)

Oatmeal, steel-cut .... 5 g per cup

Blackberries .... 8 g per cup

Nuts (i.e. almonds, pistachios) .... 3 g per oz

Apple .... 4 g per 1 medium apple with skin

Strawberries .... 3 g per cup

Pumpkin seeds .... 5 g per oz

Prunes .... 9 g per cup

Prune juice .... 3 g per cup

Temporary low-fiber diets

Depending on medical history and the type of surgery, some people may need to temporarily limit or avoid fibrous foods after surgery—make sure to speak with your healthcare team to see if you have any postoperative dietary restrictions. If you need to follow a low fiber diet, choose white grains instead of wheat, rye, barley, pumpernickel, etc. Avoid raw vegetables and choose cooked vegetables that are soft—if you can cut them with a fork, they are likely to be low enough in fiber. Choose ripe fruit that you can take the skin off of, like a banana or melon. Drink pulp-free juice—except for prune juice, which you shouldn't drink at all. You will also want to avoid nuts and seeds, but smooth/creamy peanut butter or almond butter is fine.

Consume Enough Calories, Protein, and Fluids

If you have decreased appetite after surgery and are eating less than usual, it's important to ensure you're still consuming enough calories, protein, and fluids to support wound healing. The amount of calories, protein, and fluids you need depends on many factors, including body size, activity, medical history, the type of surgery you had, and the size of your incision(s). Your registered dietitian can help determine how much nutrition you need and help you create strategies and meal plans to reach your goals.

Protein-rich foods include eggs, fish, chicken, meat, beans, lentils, cheeses, and other dairy such as yogurt. Did you know Greek yogurt is strained? This gives it a thicker consistency and more protein per ounce than most non-Greek yogurts.

Some protein-packed foods and the grams (g) of protein per serving

Egg.. 6 g per large egg

Fish ....20 g per 3 oz

Chicken .... 27 g per 3 oz breast

Greek yogurt.................................17 g per ¾ cup

Cottage cheese ....13 g per ½ cup

Chickpeas ....7 g per ½ cup

Cheese.. 7 g per oz

Edamame...17 g per ½ cup

Nuts... 7 g per oz

Peanut butter...............................9 g per 2 tablespoons

Lentils...9 g per ½ cup

Beans ....8 g per ½ cup

Barley..5 g per ¼ cup (dry)

Quinoa ....6 g per ¼ cup (dry)

Section Two

Surgery

Chapter 4

What to Expect on the Day of Your Surgery

Your surgery can take place in one of two types of settings: outpatient and inpatient. The type of setting will play a role in the outcome of your surgery day. Outpatient means that the procedure will be done in an office, surgery center, or hospital setting; you are typically discharged and sent home on the same day the surgery is performed. Inpatient means that you will stay in the hospital after the surgery for one or more days. A couple days before your surgery, it is extremely important to confirm the following:

- The type of surgery you are having
- The location of where the surgery will take place
- If your surgery will be an inpatient or outpatient procedure
- If you will be staying overnight
- The date and time of your surgery (Sometimes it is not possible to know the exact time of the surgery, for various reasons, until the day before. If this is the case, you will need to find out when you will be notified of the time.)

The Night before Surgery

All surgery procedures require a certain fasting regimen (no food or drink). Ask your doctor how long you need to fast prior to surgery. Some surgeries only require an eight-hour fast, but others may require a 12-hour or longer fast. Be sure to get specific instructions on your fasting program well ahead of your scheduled surgery date.

If you are diabetic, ask your doctor when it's safe for you to begin to fast without affecting your blood sugar.

Following your fast strictly is important because if you don't you can vomit when under anesthesia—and this can be deadly. If you don't follow the recommended time without eating, the doctor or anesthesiologist could cancel the surgery right before it is scheduled to start, due to high safety risks. So follow their directions carefully!

Shower prior to surgery to remove bacteria from your body. Some doctors will give you a specific type of antibacterial soap to wash with. Do not apply perfumes, lotions, creams, moisturizers, or makeup. For procedures requiring general anesthesia, it is recommended to remove nail polish or acrylic nails for proper monitoring of oxygen saturation.

The Day of Your Surgery

Clothing

On that day do not wear jewelry. Wear loose-fitting clothes that are comfortable and will keep you relaxed. Do not wear clothes that go over your head. A full buttoned or zippered shirt will be easiest to get back on after your procedure.

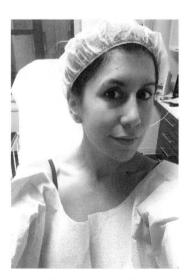

Photo 1: Pre-op selfie

Check-In

Make sure you have a friend or family member to escort you to the office or hospital. They should confirm the time you are to be picked up. It is mandatory that you have someone escort you home after surgery—otherwise you will not be released.

When you arrive, check in with the nurse or receptionist and they will escort you to the preparation area. You will change into a gown and, often, also a hat to cover your hair. Depending on the area of your procedure, you may be asked to put on disposable underwear.

Consent Forms

To have surgery, you need to sign a consent form. Signing the consent form shows that you know what the surgery is for, understand what the benefits and risks are, and allow the doctors and other hospital staff to proceed with the surgery. You may be asked to sign a release form so your doctor can use your pictures for learning purposes. You always have the right to refuse disclosure of any information or pictures.

Within the forms you sign, you will be informed of your rights under the Health Insurance Portability and Accountability Act (HIPAA) of 1996. HIPAA addresses the privacy and security of your health care data. If you have any questions regarding your HIPAA rights, please visit the website of the US Department of Health and Human services: www.HHS.gov.

Pre-Surgical Markings

At this time the doctor will meet with you. He will speak with you and mark your body prior to surgery. Surgical marking is the norm in plastic surgery and is part of the surgery plan.

How do I explain it in layman's terms? Okay, it was like when I was rushing my sorority. We heard all these rumors that girls were forced to stand in the middle of the room and someone circles your fat for the rest of the pledges to see. Luckily that didn't happen to me when I was pledging a sorority, but that's kind of what it is like to have your surgical area marked—except it is just you and the doctor.

The surgeons do this because pre-planning is necessary due to the nature of the operation. The surgical incisions are critical to optimizing how well hidden the final scars will ultimately be.

The surgeon also may do a mental walk-through which reviews the sequence of specific surgical maneuvers.

Surgical marks will help alleviate your fears because they show attention to detail and allow the doctor to make last-minute changes. Prior to liposuction, the markings show where the most fat needs to be removed. Surgical marking has always been and will always be a critical part of the plastic surgery process. It is a practice that has been standard in plastic surgery ever since plastic surgery started being performed.

Before other types of surgery, a doctor will mark the area on the patient with his name to prevent operating on the wrong area. For example, if you were having a knee replacement on the right knee, the doctor will often sign his name on the right leg to prevent operating on the wrong leg. Wrong-site surgery is very rare in plastic surgery because of all the pre-surgical markings.

Here are examples of pre-surgical markings:

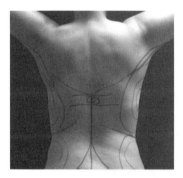
Photo 2: Pre-surgical markings (back view)

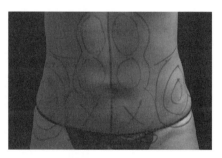
Photo 3: Pre-surgical markings (front view)

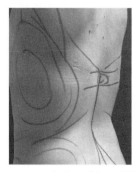
Photo 4: Pre-surgical markings (side view)

Meet the Anesthesiologist

After you are all marked up, you will meet your anesthesiologist, who will recheck your medical history and test results. He or she will also re-ask you some medical questions. It is important that the anesthesiologist be aware of all prescription, non-prescription and street drugs, i.e. heroin or cocaine, you are taking. As mentioned before, these drugs can interact with the anesthesia and cause a bad reaction—or death. Inform the doctor if you have loose teeth or crowns because if they come loose during surgery, you could choke on them. A detailed history will ensure a safe surgery.

The anesthesiologist will be in charge of administering and monitoring your anesthesia care throughout the surgery. Though you may still be able to walk, you might be taken to surgery in a wheelchair or on a stretcher for the safest transportation. Before going to the operating room, you may be taken to a surgery waiting area, called a holding area. Depending on the hospital's policy, family or friends may be allowed to come with you into the holding area. In the surgery holding area, you may see other patients and a lot of activity. From the surgery holding area, you will then be moved to the operating room, also known as the OR.

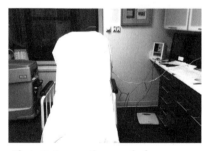

Photo 5: Preparation area before surgery

When I was going in for my surgery, I had a long talk with the anesthesiologist. One of my concerns was that when I had anesthesia in the past (had my tonsils removed), I woke up from surgery extremely nauseated—and then vomited. That was the worst feeling in the world—worse than any pain. I did not want to feel that nauseated again. I also told him that in the past when I had anesthesia, I was very sensitive to it—I was told this by other anesthesiologists, meaning that the nurses had a hard time waking me up from anesthesia. The doctor said this was very helpful information. He changed my anesthesia cocktail by adding in extra anti-nausea medication and he did not use as high a dosage of anesthesia.

In the Operating Room

Once you are brought into the operating room, your team of medical doctors and nurses will begin to prep you for the procedure. If anesthesia has not already been started in the holding area, it will be started in the operating room.

Types of Anesthesia

The choice of anesthesia to be used on you is made by the anesthesiologist. Prior to surgery, each patient is interviewed and examined by the anesthesiologist, who then tailors the plans for the anesthesia procedure.

The doctor will always choose the safest type of anesthesia for you. People commonly believe that local and regional are the safest form of anesthesia, but this is not always true. For major surgery, general anesthesia is a safer route. Regional anesthesia is not always 100 percent effective. If regional anesthesia fails after the surgery has begun, switching to a different form of anesthesia can be dangerous.

General anesthesia

General anesthesia is a treatment that renders you unconscious during the surgery. It may be used for any type of surgery and is used for more major procedures. You won't feel or remember anything that happens.

To achieve the right effects, the anesthesiologist often combines sleep-inducing agents, i.e. hypnotics, with analgesics, i.e. medications that relieve pain but don't block other sensations, and muscle relaxants. Many of these medications are administered through an intravenous catheter, called an IV, which is placed in your vein before surgery. The anesthesiologist often starts with a medication to relieve anxiety. The sleep you experience under general anesthesia is different from regular sleep. A body that is sedated by general anesthesia does not respond to pain signals or surgical manipulations. To begin the process of general anesthesia, the anesthesiologist will give you medication through your IV that will make you fall asleep before you can count to 100. After you fall asleep, a tube may be placed in your throat to help you continue breathing easily throughout your surgery. This tube is called an endotracheal (ET) tube.

Regional anesthesia

Regional anesthesia is the administration of some type of nerve block, which makes a particular body area numb and insensitive to pain. For example, regional anesthesia would make an entire leg numb. Along with the numbness, you would experience temporary paralysis of the leg as well.

During regional anesthesia, you are awake or in a very light sleep. Light sleep is induced to relieve anxiety for some people. Patients that undergo regional anesthesia may occasionally need the doctor to switch to general anesthesia during the surgery.

There are different types of regional anesthesia, i.e. spinal block, epidural block, Beer's block, and ankle block. Spinal anesthesia involves the injection of a small amount of local anesthetic directly into the cerebrospinal fluid surrounding the spinal cord. This may cause a drop in blood pressure but that is easily treated. Epidural anesthesia involves the injection of a large volume of local anesthetic directly into the space surrounding the epidural sac that contains the spinal fluid—the anesthetic does not go into the spinal fluid. Pain relief occurs more slowly but is less likely to produce blood pressure drops. Also, the block can be safely maintained for long periods, even days if necessary! Nerve blocks involve the injection of an anesthetic into the area around the nerve that runs to a particular region of the body, preventing the nerve from carrying nerve impulses such as pain to the brain.

Local anesthesia

Local anesthesia is the injection of a nerve-blocking medication, i.e. lidocaine, directly into the skin or muscle of a small area of the body. This is commonly used for very minor procedures such as removal of a mole from the skin.

Conscious sedation

This is the induction of light sleep, meaning that the cerebral cortex is asleep and the patient is not conscious. However, the sleep is not so deep that it stops brainstem activity. This means that the respiratory centers, which are in the brainstem, are still functioning and the patient is breathing on their own. And the patient is not paralyzed and can still move on their own—and may be quickly awakened.

Conscious sedation is commonly used in combination with regional and local anesthesia. The major disadvantage of this technique is that if the patient stops breathing, the anesthesiologist does not have control of the airway until an ET tube is placed—an emergency situation.

Vital signs

Anesthesiologists monitor your vital signs throughout your surgical procedure. You can relax in the knowledge that you will be closely monitored in the operating room by the anesthesiologist. Your anesthesiologist will continually monitor your pulse, heart rhythm, blood pressure, respiration, and the oxygen level in your blood. They will give you any necessary medications, fluids, or blood products during your surgery.

Equipment

The following is typical equipment used to monitor your vital signs:

- A sphygmomanometer is a blood pressure cuff, used to monitor your blood pressure.
- A pulse oximeter, is either a finger clip or sticky pad, used to measure your blood oxygen level.

- Electrodes are placed on your chest to monitor your heart rate and other aspects of your electrocardiogram, also known as an ECG or EKG.

Oxygen and Fluids

During any type of surgery, it is always important that you as the patient are getting enough oxygen and proper amounts of fluids. Oxygen may be given during surgery in one of three ways:

1. Through an endotracheal (ET) tube in your throat
2. By flow through a face mask
3. Through a nasal cannula, a small tube placed just inside your nose

Fluids and medications are given though your intravenous (IV) line as needed. As with all medications, some anesthetics may interact with other medications. When this happens, the effects of one or both of the drugs may change or the risk of side effects may be greater. Anyone who receives a regional or local anesthetic should let the doctor know all other drugs he or she is taking including prescription drugs, nonprescription drugs, and street drugs, i.e. cocaine, marijuana, and heroin, to name a few.

Once you are sound asleep and your vitals are stable, your surgery will begin. If general anesthesia is not being used, you may be given a pill to relax you prior to the application of local or regional anesthesia.

Here is an example of what the inside of an operating room looks like:

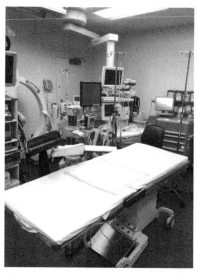

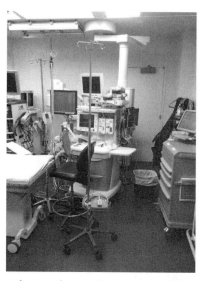

Photo 6: A typical operating room set-up   Photo 7: The anesthesiologist's station

Your surgery begins!

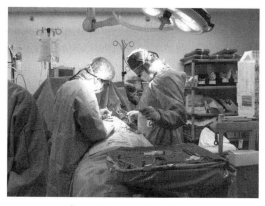

Photo 8: Surgery is underway

Recovery Room

Congratulations! Your surgery is now over! Once the surgery is over, you will be taken to a recovery area or room. This is where your sedation wears off and you slowly awaken. A nurse will be present to monitor your vital signs and to make sure you are not vomiting or in pain. If you feel any pain or experience nausea, you will be given medication through your IV.

You may feel groggy coming out of anesthesia—this is normal. Many people experience side effects following general anesthesia. These side effects typically appear within a few hours after the surgery and usually resolve themselves on their own but can last for several days. The feeling of a sore throat or dry throat is typically the first thing patient's notice. This is usually the result of the ET tube used to help the patients breathe during the surgery, but sometimes it can be due to the relatively dry air in the OR. People also report feeling dehydrated and nauseated, and sometimes feeling like they are hungover. They also may report headaches and pain in their muscles or joints. These side effects are generally no worse in intensity than symptoms of a cold or flu.

Once the sedation wears off, you will become more alert. Then the nurse will have you try to take sips of water and use the bathroom. Your doctor will usually expect that you be able to urinate and walk before you can be discharged home.

When I first came out of surgery, I was really groggy. I had to adjust to my surroundings and remember where I was. Once my eyes starting adjusting, I saw a sweet nurse in front of me. She was saying, "Hi… it's all done now…your surgery went great…I am here to help you. Do you have pain? Are you nauseated?" I was able to whisper "No," but as I spoke, I noticed my throat was sore. I remember feeling really happy that I wasn't in pain or nauseated, but then I did start to feel something—like I couldn't breathe. I told the nurse, "I am having a hard time breathing." She immediately came over and asked me a million questions and checked my vital signs. She said my oxygen level was in the acceptable range, but she wanted to make sure. She called the anesthesiologist back in to examine me. He said I was okay—but he stayed with me for a while to make sure. They had me sit up at the edge of the bed and take deep breaths. I started to cough, I felt something stuck in my chest, but I couldn't cough it out. The nurse then started doing chest PT—percussions on my back with cupped hands—to help me clear my airway. After the deep breaths and chest PT, I started coughing—and coughing! I coughed up thick bloody gunk—phlegm! It was gross—but then I could breathe better. The nurse said some bloody phlegm was normal because of the breathing tube. Another part of the reason I felt I couldn't breathe was because the garment was so constricting—it felt really, really tight, but it needs to be tight! The nurse gave me a little medication for anxiety, and then I felt calmer—that always makes things better!

The following pictures were taken immediately after I woke up from surgery. Photo 9 is when I first sat up after surgery, at the edge of the bed, to breathe better. My vital signs were monitored and then the nurse did chest physical therapy (PT). You can see that I am wearing a full upper-body garment.

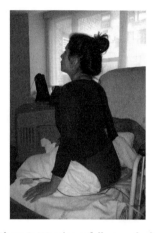

Photo 9: Wearing a full upper-body garment in the recovery room

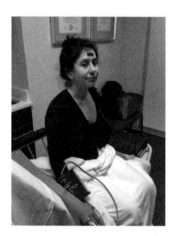

Photo 10: I've looked and felt better than this—eek!

Mobility after Surgery

Getting in and out of bed can seem like a simpler idea than it is—especially after abdominal or breast surgery. Many say that getting in and out of bed after surgery is surprisingly extremely difficult.

Sitting up may be tricky, so here are a few pointers on the best way to sit up. If you just have had abdominal or breast surgery, it will be difficult or uncomfortable to sit straight up from a lying-down position. When treating patients in the hospital, physical therapists—like me!—instruct patients on how to more easily get in and out of bed using a log-roll technique.

Getting out of bed

1. Roll over onto your side.
2. Bend your knees until your legs are hanging over the side of the bed.
3. Use your arms to lift your upper body up so that you are sitting on the edge of the bed.
4. Push off with your arms to help you stand up.

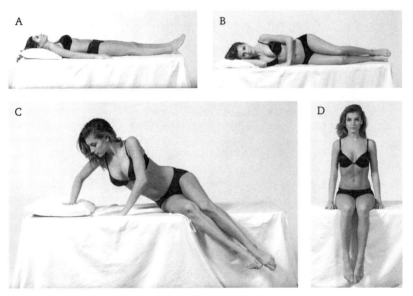

Photos 11A-D: *The log roll technique*

Once you've propped yourself up on the edge of the bed, *do not* immediately stand up and begin walking. The first time you sit up, you may experience a drop in blood pressure, feel dizzy, and/or experience increased discomfort. Sit with your legs dangling over the edge of the bed and pump your ankles, so your body can become adjusted to the upright position. These are very effective and important techniques that you'll be using in the weeks ahead so take your time and get the hang of it.

Now that you've successfully gotten yourself out of bed, eventually you will need to get back into it. Here is a way to get back into bed more easily and with minimal pain.

Getting into bed

1. Sit on the edge of your bed.
2. Start by coming down on to your forearm.
3. Gently swing your legs back onto the bed.
4. Use your arms to roll over on to your back.

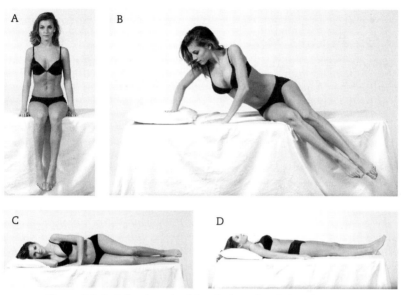

Photos 12A-D: Lying down by doing the log roll technique in reverse

Walking

It may be difficult to try to get up and walk for the first time after surgery, so ask the nurse to help you. To prevent you from falling, the nurse will walk with you until you feel steady. Walking may be too much for you immediately after surgery, so you may be assisted to a chair as the first step. Remember, drains to collect fluid from your incision and/or a Foley catheter to collect your urine may still be attached to you, so be mindful that these have to come along with you when you get out of bed! Small drains can be pinned, with a safety pin, onto your gown or clothing. If you still have a Foley catheter, you or the nurse will have to hold the bag as you walk.

Getting Discharged Home

After outpatient surgery, once the nurse and doctor determine you are stable, you will be discharged home. After inpatient surgery, your doctor may want you to stay in the hospital overnight or for a few days. On the day you are discharged, your nurse will give you specific discharge instructions appropriate to your surgery. Most of your discharge instructions will be addressed in this book, but since some are tailored to your particular surgery, it's important to pay attention when your nurse goes over all your discharge instructions.

When you are discharged, the person you have designated to pick you up will be present to help you get home. You might still be drowsy or unsteady from the anesthesia, or not back to full strength yet, so make sure your escort is holding your hand or otherwise guarding you when you stand and walk, to prevent you from falling.

The Car Ride Home

It's a good idea to protect the seat you will be sitting on with towels or a protective disposable pad. It is possible that you will leak on your way home. You don't want to ruin the seat.

Next, getting into the car may be tricky. A tip for getting into the car is to first move the passenger-side seat back, so there is ample leg space. Next, turn your body around so your back faces the side of the seat, and begin by sitting. Hold onto the frame of the car. If you only hold onto the car door, it could move or swing shut as you are sitting and you fall. Lastly, have your escort help bring your legs into the car, one at a time.

If you have had abdominal or breast surgery, wearing a seatbelt might feel painful but since it's still important to be safe, place a thin pillow or folded towel between your chest/abdomen and the seat belt.

Before I had my surgery, I did not think about preparing the car at all. Thank goodness there were makeshift supplies in the trunk—extra doggy wee-wee pads from taking the dog to the vet, plus towels.

Otherwise the car seat would have been ruined from the bloody drainage leaking out of my incision sites.

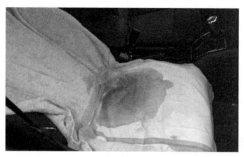

Photo 13: The car seat after my ride home from surgery

Once you arrive home, you can exit the car in a similar way. Begin by bringing your legs out of the car, with help from your escort if needed. Then have your escort take one of your hands and use your other hand to hold onto the door frame of the car—not the car door which might swing and push you off balance. Pull yourself into a standing position and let your escort help you as you walk. If you have to manage stairs to get into your home, take your time and place one hand on the railing. Allow your escort to assist you by holding your other arm or hand.

Now You're Home

Once you are home, do not perform any strenuous activities. This means not lifting anything heavier than a gallon of milk, about five pounds. It's a good idea before surgery to make arrangements to have housework done for you after surgery for a while, so you won't be tempted to redecorate or start spring-cleaning when you arrive home! Your home should already be prepared for your recovery, with necessary supplies and space already set up.

Immediately following surgery, even after you are back at home, you want to get plenty of rest. Relax on the couch or your bed, dim the lights, put on some soothing music, and start sleeping. Plan to rest and relax for the entire afternoon and evening of the day you return home. Most people still feel the effects of the anesthesia and procedure—and easily sleep for most of the first day back home.

After you are home, rest up! It's time to begin the first day of recovery for a new and improved you!

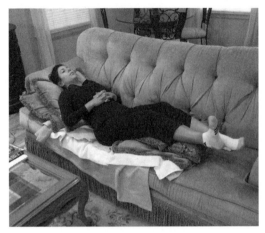

Photo 14: Resting after returning home from surgery

Section Three
Recovery After Surgery

Chapter 5

Now You Are Home...What to Do?

Get Plenty of Rest

Before surgery, you should have made arrangements for a ride home and to have someone stay with you at home, at least for the first day and night. Before surgery, you should also have made arrangements to have housework done for you for a while after your procedure. Don't be tempted to redecorate or start spring-cleaning when you arrive home! Do not perform any strenuous activities—this means do not lift anything heavier than five pounds, i.e. a gallon of milk. That's a rule!

Your home should already be prepared for your recovery with all necessary supplies and spaces already set up. Immediately following your return home from surgery, you want to get plenty of rest. Plan to rest and relax the afternoon and evening of your first day home. Most people are still feeling the effects of the anesthesia and will sleep for most of their first day home.

After surgery remember to keep the menu light. Some doctors will keep you on a liquid diet for the first postoperative meal. (No *sodium* soup is a good option). This is so you, and your stomach, can have a chance to recover.

Even after minor surgery, you may feel drowsy and tired for a number of hours. Getting in and out of bed may serve as a challenge, especially after abdominal or breast surgery. Physical therapists teach their patients how to get in and out of bed without putting strain on the abdominal muscles, using the following methods.

How to Get into Bed

1. Start by sitting on the edge of the bed.
2. Then lean down onto your forearm closest to the head of the bed.
3. Gently swing your legs onto the bed.
4. Use your arms to roll over on to your back.

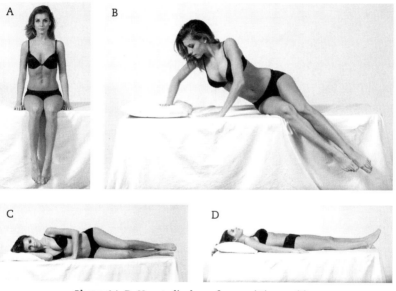

Photos 1A-D: How to lie down from a sitting position

How to Get Out of Bed

1. Roll over onto your side.
2. Bend your knees and then bring your legs over the edge of the bed.
3. Then use your arms to push yourself to a seated position.
4. Push off with your hands on the bed, to help stand up.

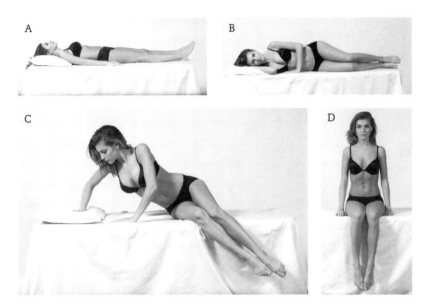

Photos 2A-D: How to sit up from a lying position

Walking after Surgery is Necessary!

After your surgery your body will begin healing. No matter what plastic surgery procedure you have, your body will go through the inflammatory process. As a result, your body will react by producing and sending increased fluid to the surgical area in order to take away waste, restore damaged cells affected by the surgery, and heal your body.

Walking will allow your body to assist with the movement of the extra fluid, which will restore order in your body and heal your body quicker. Walking is a muscle-pumping activity, which promotes the movement of fluid within your body. With each step that you take, your calf and thigh muscles will squeeze the veins in your legs, and this will help push blood, along with other fluids and wastes, back to your heart so your heart can pump them to your kidneys and liver to be eliminated.

The great thing about walking is that you can do it anywhere and anytime! You can choose to walk outdoors or indoors, depending on the weather. You can use gym tracks, parks, high-school tracks—I personally loved healing my body walking through malls. OMG, I sound like my grandmother, but that's okay, it works. Right after surgery I tell patients to avoid walking on a treadmill. I prefer you maintain your own pace at which you feel comfortable—not having the treadmill dictate the speed. I have had a couple patients fall off the treadmill post surgery; no one needs a broken hip after liposuction—ain't nobody got time for that.

When prepping for your walks, make sure to choose a place to walk that is not too cold or too hot because extreme temperatures may affect your body's response. If it's too hot, an increase in body temperature generally increases blood flow throughout, which will cause you to swell more.

Keep in mind that after certain surgeries you may find it more difficult to walk and exercise due to pain and range of motion restrictions. For example, after an abdominoplasty or tummy tuck, standing up straight may be difficult at first because the surgeon has tightened all of the excess abdominal skin. You should not forcibly stand up straight for the first week or two, depending on how much the doctor tightened the area. Keep a slight flexed posture and then gradually stand up straighter after the first week. As with any surgery, please follow any precautions or restrictions that your surgeon gives you at the time of discharge from the hospital or office.

I recommend that even before your surgery, you start a walking program—this will allow you to set a pace and distance that you are comfortable with. You want to achieve a moderate pace that you can perform several times a day.

Rating of Perceived Exertion

The intensity of your walking can be monitored, and altered, by using the Rating of Perceived Exertion (RPE). This scale rates the intensity of your exercise—in this case, walking—from zero to 10. A moderate pace is equivalent to a rating of four to seven on this exertion scale. As a rule of thumb, if you can talk but not sing during an activity, it is a moderate-intensity activity.

RPE SCALE	
0	nothing at all
0.5	very, very weak
1	very weak
2	weak
3	moderate
4	somewhat strong
5	strong
6	
7	very strong
8	
9	
10	very, very strong
Maximal	

Photo 3: Rating scale for perceived exertion

By establishing a solid walking program, you are ensuring that your successful surgery will remain a success as you recover!

Walking Chart

Here is a sample graph for your walking program that I came up with for you to fill in every day.

Here's a sample walking program which you can use as a guide

	Minutes Walked	Distance Walked	Rate of Perceived Exertion (0–10 scale)
Day 1			
Day 2			
Day 3			
Day 4			
Day 5			
Day 6			

Photo 4: A daily way to keep track of walking progress

How to Prevent a Blood Clot after Surgery

What is a Blood Clot?

A blood clot is a mass of clumped together blood, or platelets, in the blood vessel. It is a serious condition that can be deadly. Having any type of surgery puts a person at risk for getting a blood clot. Most people do not think this includes plastic surgery—but it does! A person who has liposuction, or any other surgery, on their legs is at even a higher risk because the most common type of blood clot forms in deep veins in your legs. As a professional, I have seen patients get a blood clot after plastic surgery—but luckily the clots were all caught in time and the patients did not die.

In recent years, the Surgeon General reported 350,000 to 600,000 blood clots per year resulting in at least 100,000 deaths. Here are four things that will increase your risk for developing a blood clot:

1. Not walking regularly after surgery.
2. Having a pre-existing medical condition, such as cancer or a blood-clotting disorder.
3. The longer your surgery takes, i.e. the longer you are on the operating table.
4. Undergoing general anesthesia.

Signs You Might Have a Blood Clot

If you are experiencing any of these four warnings signs, call your doctor immediately!

1. Sudden bad pain in your calf or leg. Generally, the pain is in one calf or leg only, not both at the same time.
2. Sudden swelling in the calf or leg.
3. If the calf or leg begins to turn a reddish-blue color.
4. If the calf or leg feels very warm or hot.

Simple Test for a Blood Clot

The clinical test for a blood clot in the leg is called the Homan's sign. This test is performed by flexing the leg at the hip and knee, then the tester quickly dorsiflexes the ankle and palpates the calf. Pain in the calf is a positive sign, which may indicate that the person has a blood clot. A positive Homan's sign may mean a blood clot, but a negative doesn't mean there is not a blood clot. If you think you might have a blood clot, call your doctor. This test is not 100 percent accurate—so you should always call your doctor if you think you might have the signs of a blood clot, even if the Homan's sign is negative!

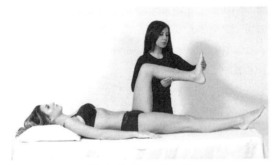

Photo 5: Homan's test

Signs that a Blood Clot May Have Gone to Your Lungs

If a blot clot in your leg gets loose from the vein, it can travel through your bloodstream to your lungs or other organs. When it travels to your lungs, it is called a pulmonary embolism—this is serious, as it often causes sudden death!

Contact your doctor immediately if you notice any of these symptoms:

Stabbing chest pain

Shortness of breath

Rapid or irregular heart beat

Dizziness

Fainting

Excessive sweating

Sudden and unexplained anxiety

Excessive coughing

Coughing up blood

Four Ways to Prevent a Blood Clot

You should do all four: wear compression stockings, change your body position frequently, pump your ankles, and walk, walk, walk!

1. Compression stockings

Compression stockings are designed to prevent blood clots. It is recommended that after surgery, you wear compression stockings, also called anti-embolism stockings, until you are moving normally again, consistently.

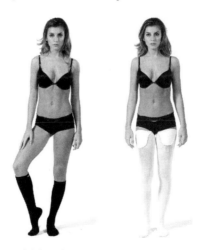

Photo 6: Knee-high and over-the-knee compression stockings

2. Change your position

Change the position of your body at least every two hours, 24/7. Obviously it is a lot harder to have control over this in your sleep, but be aware and make an effort. Move from your back to your side, then to your other side. Use pillows as needed to protect your surgical incision.

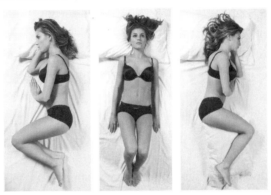

Photo 7A-C: Changing position frequently is important to prevent blood clots

3. Ankle pumps

Ankle pumps are one of the most important exercises for patients to perform immediately after any surgery! Routinely, swelling tends to pool in the lower leg and ankles after surgery. When your muscles contract, they apply pressure to the veins in the lower legs to pump blood and lymph fluid out of the area. This will help prevent blood clots!

Move your foot up and down like you're pumping a gas pedal, by alternately contracting your calf and shin muscles. Perform ankle pumps in bed every two hours by bending your ankles up and down for a few minutes, alternating your feet.

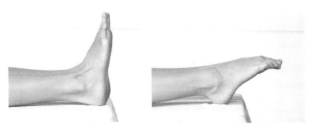

Photo 8A-B: Ankle pumps

4. Walking

Make sure to get up and walk every few hours starting immediately after surgery unless your doctor gives you other instructions. The general rule of thumb is that a patient should be getting out of bed to walk to the bathroom as soon as is necessary, starting in the recovery room.

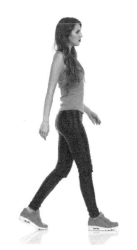

Photo 9: Begin walking as soon as possible after surgery (courtesy of shutterstock.com)

How to Prevent Pneumonia after Surgery

1. Deep Breathing

Deep breathing keeps your lungs healthy while you heal. Many patients feel weak and sore after surgery, so taking big breaths can be uncomfortable. However, if you do not work on deep breathing after surgery, you may develop lung problems, most commonly *pneumonia*.

A device called an *incentive spirometer* can help you take deep breaths correctly. You use an incentive spirometer by placing the tip of the hose in your mouth. Next, you suck in slowly, as if you were sucking a thick milkshake through a straw. Make sure to inhale for at least a count of eight seconds. You then exhale slowly, emptying the air out of your lungs.

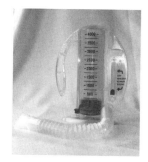

Photo 10: One type of incentive spirometer

If you do not own an incentive spirometer, you can still practice deep breathing on your own. Perform ten repetitions of slow deep inhaling and exhaling every two hours. Place your hands on your stomach, then your ribs, and breathe deeply, feeling your stomach wall and rib cage move. It's not enough to just move your rib cage. Breathe in through your nose (like your are smelling flowers) and out through pursed lips (like you are blowing out birthday candles). Breathe in and out for a count of eight seconds in each direction.

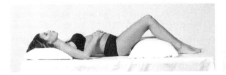

Photo 11: Deep inhale.

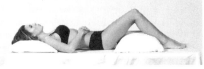

Photo 12: Deep exhale.

2. Coughing

Many patients avoid coughing because it can be very painful—but you must cough enough to prevent lung complications. If it hurts when you cough, you should brace your incision by hugging a small pillow to the area when you cough, applying gentle but firm pressure. If your incision is on your chest, i.e. breast augmentation, you would hug a pillow to your chest directly over your incision. If your incision is on your abdomen, i.e. tummy tuck, you would hug a pillow to your incision at your pelvis. If no pillow is available, you can use your hands to brace your incision—the pillow is primarily for comfort. Even if your incision is not on your chest or abdomen, bracing may help with pain control.

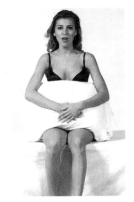

Follow these tips and you will set yourself up on the road to recovery!

Photo 13: Bracing with a pillow when coughing

Chapter 6
Warning Signs of a Problem During Recovery

It is normal to have some side effects after surgery, i.e. pain, discomfort, swelling, and bruising. But you have to be aware of and pay attention to some warning signs that are not normal. If you experience any of the following symptoms, contact your doctor immediately.

General Warning Signs

Symptoms

Body temperature over 100.4 degrees Fahrenheit, with or without chills

Fainting

Shortness of breath

Severe/worsening fatigue

Coughing up or vomiting blood

Excessive amounts of bleeding

Excessive amounts of swelling

Severe confusion or delirium

Inability to urinate for 24 hours or have a bowel movement for more than several days

Inability to walk or collapsing while walking

If you have any side effects to medications, i.e. rash, nausea, headache, or vomiting

Rapid heart rate (over 100 bpm)—normal resting heart rate or pulse for adults is 60–100 beats per minute.

Intense Pain or Decreased Sensation

Chest pain that is sharp and shooting or feels like severe pressure. If you experience severe pressure or sharp, shooting pain in your chest, call your doctor or 911 immediately.

Severe or increased pain anywhere in your body not relieved by medication.

Unexplained severe pain and swelling in your calf or leg, which can be a sign of a blood clot.

Some numbness at the surgical site is normal, but loss of feeling or motion anywhere in your body might be a sign of nerve damage.

Incision Problems

If your incision is warm, red, swollen, and tender, you may have an infection.

As infection spreads, you may develop a fever, chills, and swollen glands.

Excessive pus, i.e. yellow or green drainage, coming from the incision

A bad odor coming from your incision

The sides of the incision separate or open up

Tissue Problems

Necrosis

If the surgery site does not get enough blood supply, the tissue may turn black or begin to die. This is called necrosis.

Hematoma

A hematoma is a pocket of blood formed by when blood leaks out into tissue. It can look somewhat like a blood blister.

Seroma

A seroma is a pool of fluid that develops in tissue after surgery. It usually develops in the stomach area, most often the lower stomach. You can tell you have a seroma because when you touch it, you see a "waterbed effect." You can see the fluid underneath moving in a wave-like pattern. It is not dangerous but can lead to an infection.

Surgery-Specific Warning Signs

Abdominoplasty (Tummy Tuck) or Body Lift

See general warning signs above.

Look for areas that have opened along the incision line.

An infection along the incision may cause redness, swelling, pain, or foul-smelling drainage.

Some clear or blood-tinged drainage is expected but excessive amounts of bleeding are not normal.

Pain that is more than your basic stomach ache or soreness.

The most serious sign of a complication of abdominal surgery is severe abdominal pain.

Breast Augmentation

See general warning signs above.

One breast is more swollen than the other, which may be due to excessive bleeding.

One breast sits higher than the other, which may be due to excessive bleeding or the implant shifting out of its pocket.

Numbness in the arm may be due to blood or fluid

compressing the nerves that go down your arm—this can be a serious complication.

Sudden and drastic color change in tissue, whether lighter or darker, can be caused by a serious complication.

One breast flattens, or is significantly smaller, can be a sign of a rupture.

Severe pain in the chest area—but remember that mild to moderate soreness is normal and expected.

Implant extrusion: Extrusion means the implant is literally coming out of the body. The skin breaks down and the implant pops out.

Capsular contracture: A combination of pain, hardening, and stiffness in the breast is an indication of capsular contracture, which occurs when scar tissue forms around the implant.

Breast Lift

See general warning signs above.

One breast is more swollen than the other, which may be due to excessive bleeding.

One breast is much larger than the other, which may be due to excessive bleeding.

One breast sits higher than the other, which may indicate excess bleeding.

Numbness in the arm may be due to blood or fluid compressing the nerves that go down your arm—this can be a serious complication.

Sudden and drastic color change in tissue, whether lighter or darker, can be caused by a serious complication.

Breast Reduction

See general warning signs above.

One breast is more swollen than the other, which may be due to excessive bleeding.

One breast sits higher than the other, which may be due to excessive bleeding.

Numbness in the arm may be due to blood or fluid compressing the nerves that go down your arm—this can be a serious complication.

Sudden and drastic color change in tissue, whether lighter or darker, can be caused by a serious complication.

Buttock Implants

See general warning signs above.

Tightness and severe pain can be due to scar tissue forming around the implant, called capsular contraction.

Pain radiating down your leg can be a sign that the implant is pressing on the sciatic nerve, the largest nerve in your body.

Any numbness or pain in your legs.

One implant is higher than the other.

Implant extrusion: Extrusion means the implant is literally coming out of the body. The skin breaks down and the implant pops out.

Buttock Lift

See general warning signs above.

Asymmetric or flattened buttocks.

Bleeding under the skin that accumulates enough to look like a massive bruise or an area of purplish/black swelling.

Pain, swelling, fluid accumulation, and scarring.

Poor wound healing, i.e. when the wound separates and/or bleeds, and/or pus develops.

Recurrent skin loosening—this will require additional surgery.

Necrosis or skin tissue death (as described in general warnings)

Temporary or permanent change in skin sensation, i.e. numbness, loss of feeling, increased sensitivity.

Calf Augmentation

See general warning signs above.

Sharp shooting pains in the calf and heels could mean nerve damage.

Feet turning blue, with skin very cold to touch, and/or an absent pulse in the foot could be due to a block in blood flow, such as a blood clot.

Implant becomes visible due to incorrect pocket or implant placement.

Asymmetry is due to slippage of the implant.

Loss of sensation in the ankle or foot.

Cheek Implant

See general warning signs above.

The face can become uneven if the implants shift out of position.

Implant extrusion: This is rare in the face but can be caused by excessive trauma or infection. Extrusion means the implant literally comes out of the body. The skin breaks down and the implant pops out.

Signs of nerve damage: Drooling, facial droop, difficulty swallowing, difficulty chewing, loss of sensation, impaired hearing, difficulty talking, loss of taste, oversensitive hearing, and/or decreased salivation and tear production.

Retraction of the lower eyelid: Retraction means that the eyelid tucks in under the eyeball. This could cause dry and irritated eyes. It can happen if the implant was inserted through an incision in your eyelid.

Chin Augmentation

See general warning signs.

Nerve damage: The nerve that provides sensation for the lower lip, lower face, and chin area can be bruised and stretched during surgery, and even permanently damaged. If that nerve is damaged, a temporary or permanent numbness occurs in the lower lip, lower face, and chin area. This does not affect the movement of the lip in any way, but can cause difficulty drinking liquids due to lip numbness.

Bone resorption: Calcium is reabsorbed into the bloodstream when bone breaks down. In people with very thin jawbones, bone resorption can lead to jawbone fractures, which need to be surgically repaired.

Implant rejection: If your body's immune system decides that the implant is harmful, immune cells will attack the implant, which causes pain and swelling. The implant may need to be removed.

Implant movement: If the implant moves, it may interfere with the action of the muscles of the lower lip. That means you may not be able to move your mouth the same as before.

Infection: Typically, if the area gets infected, pus will develop in the space between your lower teeth and lip.

Ear Surgery (Otoplasty)

See general warning signs above.

Excessive bleeding or fluid seeping through the incisions

A severely misshapen appearance

Excessive bruising or fluid retention on one side of the face or head

Poor wound healing, i.e. when the wound separates and/or bleeds, and/or pus develops

Numbness or other changes in sensation of the ear

Change in ear color

Blood clots in the area of the ear

Asymmetrical ear appearance

Hearing loss

Eyelid Surgery (Blepharoplasty)

See general warning signs above.

Any change in vision, i.e. seeing flashing lights or loss of peripheral vision

Dry eye syndrome, which is usually temporary

Inability to close your eyes, which is usually temporary

Lower eyelid pulls down thus your eye becomes irritated

The edges of your eyelids pull inward, which may cause your eyelashes to rub against and irritate your eyeball.

Blindness, which is extremely rare

Seeing double or having blurry vision

Temporary swelling at the corners of the eyelids

Tiny whiteheads on the eyelids—don't try to squeeze them as that can cause dangerous infection and swelling.

Eye asymmetry or unevenness

Eyelid sagging

Difficulty blinking or keeping your eyes closed while asleep

Sunken eyes or hollowness under the eyes

Hematoma may cause severe pain that does not respond to medication, significant swelling of an eyelid, and/or excessive or increasing bruising of an eyelid.

Facelift (Rhytidectomy) or Neck Lift

See general warning signs above.

Excessive pain and swelling

Red areas around incisions could be due to infection

Earlobe deformity called "pixie ear"

Hair loss along the incision line or elsewhere

Signs of nerve damage include: facial drooping, i.e. around eye or mouth, difficulty swallowing or chewing, drooling, impaired sensation or numbness of parts of the face, impaired hearing, difficulty talking, loss of taste, hearing sensitivity, and decreased salivation and tear production.

Forehead or Brow Lift

See general warning signs above.

Numbness of your forehead or inability to raise your eyebrow

Facial or brow asymmetry

Poor wound healing, i.e. when the wound separates and/or bleeds, and/or pus develops

Hair loss along the incisions

Loss of eyelashes or eyebrows

Skin loss

Eye irritation or dryness

Eyelid droops or is pulled up

Skin contours are uneven

Hair Transplantation

See general warning signs above.

Hair does not grow back because hair follicles have died after being transplanted.

A patchy, unnatural-appearing hair pattern

Excessive bleeding

Inflammation or infection of the hair follicles

Shock loss, which is sudden loss of the transplanted hair, which is usually temporary

Lip Augmentation (Surgical/ Non-Injection)

See general warning signs above.

Infection, irritation, necrosis, and/or hematoma

Permanent discolorations from bruising can occur.

Granuloma formation due to severe inflammation.
A granuloma is a kind of non-cancerous lump.

Implant extrusion: This is rare in the face but can be caused by excessive trauma or infection.

Implant extrusion: means the implant literally comes out of the body. The skin breaks down and the implant pops out.

Liposuction or Lower Body Lift

See general warning signs above.

Redness, swelling, pain, and/or foul-smelling drainage around the incision indicates an infection.

Some clear or blood-tinged drainage is expected, but excessive amounts of bleeding are not normal.

Pain that is more than your basic stomach ache or soreness.

The most serious sign of a complication of abdominal liposuction is severe abdominal pain.

Pectoral Implants

See general warning signs above.

Implant shifting, i.e. one is higher than the other, or the implant shifts to the side

See warnings signs for breast implants, noting that pectoral implants rarely rupture.

Nose Surgery (Rhinoplasty)

See general warning signs above.

Pain or swelling, especially increasing after the third day after your surgery

Reddened cheeks can be a sign of infection.

Pus coming out of the nose or nose bleed

Breathing issues (nasal obstruction)

Unintentional whistling during speech or singing

The graft or implant can migrate, causing a crooked appearance.

Sinusitis, i.e. infection of the sinus cavities, can occur within weeks of rhinoplasty and is usually related to internal swelling. The symptoms of sinus infection include a lack of smell, headache, or feelings of pressure in the sinuses, nasal discharge, congestion, and bad breath. Although symptoms of sinusitis often are similar to those of the common cold, when such symptoms develop following rhinoplasty, contact your surgeon to rule out a bacterial infection.

Thigh Lift

See general warning signs above.

Changes in skin sensation such as numbness and pain

Poor wound healing

If incisions for an inner thigh lift are made too close to a woman's vagina and the skin is later closed only superficially, the appearance of a "gaping vagina" may occur.

Tissue or skin necrosis

Upper Arm Lift

See general warning signs above.

Fat necrosis, i.e. fatty tissue found deep in the skin might die

Damage to deeper structures such as nerves, blood vessels, muscles, and even your lungs

Numbness or weakness in the arm or hand

Remember!

Contact your doctor if you think something is wrong! This is very important and I promise that your doctor will not think you are crazy!

It is better to be overly cautious about your healing process rather than to ignore possibly serious symptoms. I urge you to take to heart all warning signs, and anything else unusual for your body, and contact your doctor promptly with any further questions or concerns.

Chapter 7
The Stages of Healing and Managing Pain

The human body does not recognize the difference between an injury coming from a mugger's knife or a surgeon's scalpel. Your mind may understand the difference between surgery and assault, but our body does not. It only feels pain. Your mind notices an interruption in its normal processes and responds to heal and repair itself.

Now that your surgery is over, it is important to understand that your recovery process begins immediately after surgery. You need to know what is happening to your body and what to expect in the healing process. No matter what type of surgery you have had, you can expect a few common things to happen during the healing process.

Your Body's Response to Surgery

There are four systems in your body that control your response to surgery:

1. Sympathetic Nervous System

The sympathetic nervous system prepares your body for "fight or flight." As described earlier, your body perceives surgery as a trauma. Thus, it increases heart rate and the force of heart contractions. It makes your airways dilate (widen) to make breathing easier. It causes the body to release stored energy. Insulin production is decreased and sugar production is increased because your muscles need more energy to heal. Muscular strength is increased. It also causes your palms to sweat, your pupils to dilate, and your hair to stand on end. It slows body processes that are less important in emergencies, such as digestion and urination.

2. Acute Response

Natural anti-inflammatory chemicals reduce vascular permeability. This means that small molecules like water are not permitted to flow out of the blood vessels easily. Salt and water retention occur to maintain fluid volume and cardiovascular balance. This results in swelling.

3. Endocrine Response

Many different hormones are released and some are suppressed (held back). Tissue trauma during surgery increases the production of hormones like ACTH and cortisol—which cause swelling.

4. Blood Vessels

New blood vessels are created in injured tissues after a trauma like surgery.

Three Stages of Healing

Each wound goes through certain stages of inflammation, swelling, and tissue healing. These stages often overlap and each person's time frame can be different. It is important to understand the stages of healing so you know what to expect throughout your recovery. For example, pain should be expected in the early stages but will decrease over time.

Problems can occur if proper healing is not encouraged in each phase. It is important for you to understand the process of inflammation and repair, and also how they can be influenced to speed up your recovery.

The main purpose of the two-step process of inflammation and repair is to control the effects of the injury and return the wounded tissue to a normal state. Inflammation occurs first. It disposes of foreign material and dead tissue to prepare for the repair phase. During tissue repair, new blood vessels and new tissue are produced. Later in the repair process, remodeling of the connective tissue takes place, which further increases tissue strength. The exact duration of the phases of inflammation and repair is not clear, both because the phases overlap and because it varies from one person to another.

Not all repair ends in restoration of normal tissue. Some tissues cannot regenerate completely, which is why scars form. Scar tissue provides the workable strength your body needs but is otherwise lacks function. Extensive scar tissue can be disfiguring and disrupt organ function. Factors within your control, such as smoking, affect tissue healing as well—believe me when I say that a pre-surgery cigarette is not worth the scar tissue it causes.

Stage 1. Acute Inflammatory Phase—Post-Op Days 1 to 10

This is the time right after your surgery. This phase will last several days. Inflammation begins when an injury or disease causes a disruption in the normal functions of the tissue—when the surgeon's scalpel cuts into your body during plastic surgery. Your tissue is put on the defense, and inflammation is the way your body protects itself.

The local five signs that are typical of the inflammatory process are called the cardinal signs of inflammation—pain, swelling, redness, warmth in the injured area, and loss of function. This local response is expected to be small to moderate. It's when these become severe that it's a problem.

The systemic response throughout your body to inflammation includes increased fluid outside your cells (extracellular fluid), increased swelling (edema) due to increased permeability of your blood vessels, decreased urine output and more concentrated urine, water retention and delayed water and sodium excretion, temporary slowing of metabolism followed by protein and weight loss, fats and proteins broken down to make more blood sugar, acid-base (pH) imbalance, suppression of your immune system, low tissue oxygen, and increased clotting risk. So, you can see that after surgery, a lot is going on in the area of your incision and also throughout your body.

While the initial inflammatory phase protects you, it can cause problems as well. If inflammation gets out of control, it can spread to areas that are not injured or last for periods of time longer than what is needed. Since the inflammatory phase sends out search-and-destroy cells and chemicals, it may break down some healthy tissue.

The most effective treatment at this stage is the combination of ice, compression, and lymphatic drainage massage (LDM). Used correctly, as described in detailed upcoming chapters, these will reduce swelling and stimulate the function of your lymphatic system. But first, some more information about the inflammatory response.

The inflammatory response can be decreased by the following: reducing trauma with good surgical technique, getting extra oxygen if necessary after surgery, antibiotics if needed, good wound care, compression, good nutrition, drinking water, icing, and controlling pain.

Four-part inflammatory response

Your inflammatory response is made up of vascular, hemostatic (clotting), cellular, and immune responses. Knowing about these four will give you the ability to understand exactly what is going on in your body during the healing process. This understanding should provide you with comfort and ease of mind as you undergo the temporary discomforts of healing.

1. Vascular response

Vascular changes—changes in your blood vessels—occur early in the inflammatory response. First, during margination, the blood vessel walls become lined with white blood cells which otherwise swim through the blood. The blood vessels, which initially constricted (clamped down) to limit blood flow, now dilate to increase both blood flow and hydrostatic pressure in the tissues. Thus, swelling occurs as the increased pressure moves fluid out of the blood vessels and into the tissues. At first, the lymphatic vessels—which usually easily carry fluid out of the tissues—are overwhelmed. Thus fluid backs up and even more tissue swelling occurs.

2. Hemostatic response

The hemostatic (clotting) response controls blood loss when blood vessels are ruptured. Platelets clump together and deposit the protein *fibrin*, which traps red blood cells, creating a blood clot. The fibrin also plugs up local lymphatic channels, preventing drainage of fluid from the injured area, thus keeping the inflammation localized so it doesn't spread throughout the body. When bleeding is internal and confined to a tissue or organ, a mass of clotted blood can develop. This is called a hematoma. Hematomas are like gigantic bruises and may cause pain or limit range of motion or function.

3. Cellular response

During the inflammatory process, germs and other debris are removed from the wound by white blood cells (leukocytes). This is very important because this prepares the area for tissue repair. There are several different types of leukocytes, which have different functions during different parts of the inflammatory process. Neutrophils eat germs and debris, and thus clear the wound area.

4. Immune response

In later stages of the immune response, lymphocytes supply the wound and the body with antibodies and secrete various proteins that act as enzymes to help your immune system.

Stage 2: Repair Phase — Post-Op Days 3 to 20

At some point after day three of recovery, your inflammation begins to go down and your body begins to repair the wound, resulting in a slight decrease in pain and swelling.

The first phase of tissue repair involves the epithelium, the cells that form both the skin and the connective tissue that is the cement that connects and supports all other tissues. During this phase, epithelial tissues renew themselves, and then fibroplasia takes place in the connective tissue. Fibroplasia is the process of creation of scar tissue—a type of connective tissue—to repair and re-establish the connective tissue.

Inadequate levels of nutrients, mainly vitamin C and oxygen, can lead to poor tissue formation, increased pain and increased risk of later injury.

Stage 3: Chronic Remodeling Phase — Post-Op Day 9 to 1–2 Years

This final phase of repair typically overlaps with Stage 2. It can start two to three weeks after surgery and can continue for up to two years. Remodeling phase is also known as the maturation phase. During this time dermal tissues enhance their tensile strength and non-functional fibroblasts are replaced by functional ones. Also the number of blood vessels in the affected areas decrease and recede as a result of cellular activity declining. As time passes, the scar tissue strengthens, but never to more than 70 or 80 percent of the original tissue's strength.

During this time there should be pain only felt with certain movements or positions. Movement and rehabilitation, in this phase, is essential to healing. If there is lack of movement, range of motion and strengthening, the tissue that forms is weak, disorganized and at risk for re-injury.

Risk for capsular contracture

During Stage 3, the risk for capsular contracture is greatest. Capsular contracture is the most common complication of breast augmentation surgery. Capsular contracture occurs as a result of excessive scar tissue formation around implanted foreign material. It is very important to prevent capsular contracture during the remodeling phase. Massage techniques should be used to reduce scarring and break down tissue adhesions. Massage therapy done on newly healed scar tissue can reduce and soften the build-up of tough fibrous tissue. Localized cross friction techniques will soften collagen. These techniques can also be used to reduce scar formation after surgeries such as a tummy tuck or body lift. Upcoming chapters give detailed information about massage and other ways to reduce scarring.

Pain

Immediately following any type of cosmetic surgery, as anesthesia wears off, you can expect soreness, discomfort, or pain. This is inevitable—everybody (mostly everyone) experiences some type of symptoms.

Pain is defined by the International Association for the Study of Pain (IASP) as "an unpleasant sensory and emotional experience associated with actual or potential tissue damage, or described in terms of such damage."

Perhaps you did not know that pain is actually a protective mechanism that alerts you to respond to prevent further injury. For example, if you accidentally touch a hot stovetop, your hand has "pain nerves" that relay the feeling to your brain, which triggers your hand to pull away to prevent further burning and pain. Similarly, when your tissues are disrupted by surgery, once the anesthetic wears off and you feel pain, your brain is triggered to make you aware that the surgery is over and a major change (trauma) in your body has taken place.

Pain is normal—do not be afraid of it. Learn how to cope with pain and heal it.

The Experience of Pain

The IASP's definition of pain emphasizes that pain is not really observable or measurable, but rather is a personal and subjective experience. Pain is an individual experience that can be influenced by culture, previous pain experience, belief, mood, and ability to cope. Some people have an extremely high pain tolerance and some people have difficulty dealing with the smallest amount of discomfort.

Pain is an uncomfortable experience, and therefore can result in increased heart rate and breathing rate, stress level, psychological and emotional state. Learning how to manage your pain is an essential part of your healing.

Three Pain-Producing Systems

Three of our systems interact to produce pain—sensory, motivational, and cognitive.

1. Your *sensory system* processes information about the strength, intensity, and quality of pain.
2. Your *motivational system* determines the nature of your approach-avoidance behaviors—how your body chooses to recognize and avoid pain.
3. Your *cognitive system* supervises your learned behavior concerning your experience of pain. It may block, manage, or enhance your perception of pain.

Neuroanatomy of Pain

Your body perceives pain when a stimulus, i.e. a pin prick, is sensed by nerve endings in your body's tissues. These nerve endings send this message through nerve pathways to your brain so your brain can interpret the pain and you can understand the pain.

The level of pain being sensed affects the intensity and speed with which the pain signal is relayed. Therefore, the greater the trauma, the more quickly and intensely the nerves will signal the brain.

Once the pain message reaches the brain, it is filtered to different areas of the brain and then is connected to a corresponding emotion. Recent studies suggest that in some people's brains, the connections between pain and emotion are particularly strong. These people feel pain more easily than others and can even feel pain when there is no outside trigger. Also, other factors, such as fatigue and sleep deprivation, can increase the body's sensitivity to pain, resulting in a lower pain threshold. It's good to know that researchers have found that positive thinking and a positive mindset can reduce pain.

Gate-control theory

Most explanations of pain are based on gate-control theory, which was proposed by Ronald Melzack and Patrick Wall during the early 1960s. Gate-control theory suggests that the spinal cord contains a neurological gate that either blocks pain signals or allows them to continue on to the brain. The idea is that physical pain is not a direct result of activation of pain receptor neurons, but rather pain perception is due to interaction between different nerve cells and fibers. The gate in the spinal cord operates by telling the difference between the types of nerve fibers carrying pain signals.

The gate-control theory brought about a drastic change in the field of pain management. The theory suggested that pain management could be achieved by selectively influencing the larger nerve fibers that do not carry pain stimuli, and that pain signal transmission can be influenced by emotions and thoughts. The gate-control theory paved the way for more research on cognitive and behavioral approaches to achieve pain relief.

Your Body's Response to Pain

If your body is in pain after surgery, you may display some or all of these signs:

Increased heart rate

Elevated blood pressure

Increased breathing rate

Increased blood sugar

Decreased insulin production

Sweating

Paleness or flushing

Dilated pupils

Increased secretion of stomach acid

Decreased activity in your stomach, intestines, and kidneys as blood flow is diverted away from them due to pain

Nausea and vomiting

Managing Pain

You can use all the knowledge about pain management that follows in this chapter to succeed on your journey through recovery!

Why Treat Pain?

Some people have a grin-and-bear-it attitude, and will choose to suffer through the pain. This is not always the healthiest thing to do for your body, because pain puts stress on you physically. You may be afraid of possibly getting addicted to pain medication—but pain medication is not the only treatment for pain.

Some of the benefits of treating your pain are:

Decreased pain and suffering

Decreased complications and negative physiological responses to pain

Decreased risk of developing chronic pain

Increased speed of recovery

Increased patient satisfaction

Increased productivity and quality of life

Measuring Pain Intensity

Pain assessment scales can be used to measure the intensity of pain. The National Initiative on Pain Control™ (NIPC) provides these tools to help you assess the severity and quality of your pain.

The first way of measuring pain is using the Visual Analog Pain Scale. This method rates pain on a scale of 0-10. In this scale a rating of 0 pain means no pain at all and a rating of 10 means the worst pain you have ever experienced. The numbers in between are a gradation between no pain and the worst pain of your life.

The second way of measuring pain is through the Wong Baker Faces Pain Rating Scale. The Wong-Baker Faces Pain Rating Scale is a pain scale that was developed by Donna Wong and Connie Baker. The scale shows a series of faces ranging from a happy face at zero, or "no hurt," to a crying face at 10, which represents "hurts like the worst pain imaginable". Based on the faces and written descriptions, the patient chooses the face that best describes their level of pain.

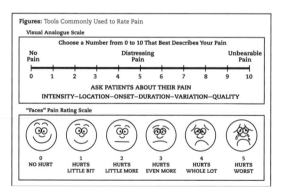

Photo 1 (top line): Visual Analog Pain Scale
Photo 1 (bottom line): Wong Baker Faces Pain Rating Scale
(courtesy of the Wong-Baker Foundation)

Pain Management

To make sure you're getting the best possible treatment for your post-surgical pain, I advise you to keep communicating with your doctor.

Pain management is a combination of medication, mind training, relaxation training, physical exercise, and alternative therapies, i.e. acupuncture.

Pain management is a branch of medicine. A typical pain management team includes one or more of the following: doctors, psychologists, physical therapists, occupational therapists, physician assistants, nurse practitioners, and clinical nurse specialists. You may also be encouraged to seek help from other professionals involved in alternative medicine, i.e. mental-health specialists, naturopathic physicians, acupuncturists, and massage therapists.

Post-surgical pain typically reaches its peak intensity two to three days after your procedure, and then gradually reduces with each passing day. This is a general estimate—your specific timeline will vary based on your procedure. Prior to surgery, speak with your doctor about the normal duration and intensity of pain expected for your procedure.

Pain Medication

A staple of medical and surgical pain management is medication. As a physical therapist, I see the impact of medication on my patients in my daily practice. I understand and observe the connection between medication side effects, mental status, and physical complaints. In most of the patients I have treated, I observed an improvement in their appearance once they stopped using prescription pain medications. Pain medications commonly cause side effects of bloating or swelling.

With any pain medication, there are common and expected side effects. In rare cases there may be more serious and potentially life-threatening complications. Ask your doctor about the symptoms of potentially serious side effects of any medication you are taking.

Common side effects of prescription pain medication

Constipation

Bloating or swelling

Fatigue and lack of energy

Nausea or vomiting

Dizziness

Feeling foggy and can't think clearly

Dry mouth

Itchiness

Irritability

Rash

Increased or decreased appetite

A drop in blood pressure

Taking or discontinuing any medication should be determined by, and discussed with, your surgeon. You should discuss with your doctor the potential benefits and side effects of the specific pain medications your doctor chooses to offer you.

Constipation and pain medication

Constipation due to pain medication seems to be one of the biggest problems for my patients. Constipation makes you feel terrible and bloated. Unfortunately, it is way too common as a side effect of pain medications.

To prevent constipation, speak to your doctor about making sure a stool softener is prescribed for you. Or, if you prefer a more natural route, I recommend fiber or fiber supplements, i.e. Miralax (polyethylene glycol), and/or prune juice, flaxseed oil, bran cereals, and herbals such as fenugreek.

Tip!

When constipated and sitting on the toilet, many people will strain. Do not do this! Straining can pop blood vessels or cause you to faint. Instead, take a deep breath and exhale while pushing—do not hold your breath!

Addiction to Pain Medication

After going through the trauma of surgery, you face another tough battle. Pain is inevitable after most surgeries. The more extensive the surgery, the longer the pain may last. Unfortunately, many of the painkillers used to treat post-surgery pain put you at risk to develop an addiction.

Anyone who takes prescription pain medication is at risk for developing an addiction. Factors like your personal life history and duration that you take the opioids, play a role in addiction development. There is no exact formula to predict who is at risk for developing a dependency. Unfortunately, these drugs are responsible for the majority of overdose deaths in the U.S today.

Before your surgery, discuss with your surgeon the plan for managing your pain after surgery. Be sure to tell your doctor if you have ever struggled with any addiction in the past—for your best outcome, it's vital that your doctor know about any past or present addiction issues you might have.

As you prepare for your surgery, start thinking about your pain management plan. Ask your doctor about how much pain you can expect to have and how long it will last. Knowing what to expect can ease your mind and make pain easier to manage. Ask the following questions about the pain medication the doctor will be prescribing for you:

Which medications will I be prescribed?
How do they work?

How long should I take them?

What are the risks for developing an addiction to them?

What signs will tell me I am getting addicted to pain meds?

Higher-risk medications

Many of the most effective painkillers available for short-term use are opioids, which all stem from the opium poppy. As street drugs, they are commonly referred to as opium or heroin. Opioids are effective painkillers, but they also give the patient the feeling of euphoria. Along with this high comes the craving to keep using it. Addiction occurs when the user develops tolerance to the drug and needs to use an ever-higher dose to get the same level of elation. Some prescription opioids are morphine, codeine, fentanyl, and oxycodone.

To prevent addiction, take your medication responsibly as prescribed and begin weaning off as soon as you can. Switch to a non-prescription medication, i.e. Extra Strength Tylenol, as soon as you can.

If you suspect you may be getting addicted to, dependent on, the pain medication, immediately discuss this with your doctor before a serious problem develops.

If you suspect you are already addicted to pain medication, contact the professionals at www.Recovery.org (1-888-249-7292) to discuss your situation.

Managing Pain with Your Mind

Pain can be reduced through learning how to relax. Relaxation training is a technique used to control pain and reduce physical and mental tension levels. Here are several relaxation techniques you can learn to help ease your pain:

Relaxation breathing

Relaxation breathing is a great way to lower stress in the body. When you breathe deeply, a message to calm down is transmitted to your brain and then relayed to the rest of your body. This results in positive changes in your body, i.e. reduced heart rate, slower breathing, and reduced blood pressure.

1. **Step 1:** Take a deep breath in through your nose for a count of four.
2. **Step 2:** Hold your breath for a count of two.
3. **Step 3:** Breathe out through your mouth for a count of eight. Repeat.

Imagine smelling flowers, then blowing out candles.

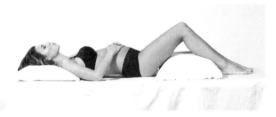

Photo 2: Relaxation breathing

Progressive muscle relaxation

Progressive muscle relaxation (PMR) is a technique for learning to monitor and control the state of muscular tension. In PMR you tense a group of muscles as you breathe in, and you relax them as you breathe out. You work on your muscle groups in a certain order.

1. **Step 1:** Assume a comfortable position. You may lie down. Loosen any tight clothing, close your eyes, and be quiet.
2. **Step 2:** Assume a passive attitude. Focus on yourself and on achieving relaxation in specific body muscles. Tune out all other thoughts.
3. **Step 3:** Tense and relax each muscle group as follows:

   - *Wrinkle your forehead and try to make your eyebrows touch your hairline for five seconds. Relax.*

   - *Close your eyes as tightly as you can for five seconds. Relax.*

   - *Draw the centers of your mouth back and grimace for five seconds. Relax. Feel the warmth and calmness in your face.*

- Extend your arms in front of you. Clench your fists tightly for five seconds. Relax. Feel the warmth and calmness in your hands.
- Extend your arms out against an invisible wall and push forward with your hands for five seconds. Relax.
- Bend your elbows. Tense your biceps for five seconds. Relax. Feel the tension leave your arms.
- Shrug your shoulders up to your ears for five seconds. Relax.
- Arch your back off the floor or off the back of your chair for five seconds. Relax. Feel the anxiety and tension disappearing.
- Tighten your stomach muscles for five seconds. Relax.
- Tighten your hip and buttock muscles for five seconds. Relax.
- Tighten your thigh muscles by pressing your legs together as tightly as you can for five seconds. Relax.
- Bend your ankles toward your body as far as you can for five seconds. Relax.
- Curl your toes as tightly as you can for five seconds. Relax.

4. **Step 4:** Focus on any muscles that may still be tense. If any muscle remains tense, tighten and relax that specific muscle three or four times.
5. **Step 5:** Fix the feeling of relaxation in your mind. Resolve to repeat the process again.

Autogenic training

Autogenic training (AT) is a relaxation technique similar to the type of meditation first introduced by German psychiatrist Johannes Schulz in the 1930s. It is believed that saying a series of mantras to yourself in a specific order can have a positive effect on your autonomic nervous system. Although less well-known than other relaxation techniques, i.e. progressive muscle relaxation and guided imagery, a study in 2002 found positive effects of autogenic training.

The basic AT exercises focus on relaxation in the body by visualizing heaviness in your body and limbs and warmth in your circulatory system. These are followed by practicing awareness of your heartbeat, breathing, abdomen, and a cool forehead. The basic practice of autogenic training consists of seven formulas that you repeat in a specific pattern. Lie down in a quiet environment, close your eyes, and repeat to yourself:

I am completely calm. (once)

My right arm is heavy. (six times)

I am completely calm. (once)

My right arm is warm. (six times)

I am completely calm. (once)

My heart beats calmly and regularly. (six times)

I am completely calm. (once)

My breathing is calm and regular—it breathes me. (six times)

I am completely calm. (once)

My abdomen is flowingly warm. (six times)

I am completely calm. (once)

My forehead is pleasantly cool. (six times)

I am completely calm. (once)

Visualization and guided imagery

Visualization and guided imagery are gentle but powerful techniques that focus and direct the imagination. They are not strictly mental activities because they involve the whole body, the emotions, and all the senses. This focus on the body makes their impact powerful.

Visualization involves visualizing something for relaxation. This may include visualizing a relaxing scene, a healing occurring, the stages of a breath, or other helpful mental images.

I tend to visualize myself in South Beach, relaxing on the

beach, with a book open and a drink in my hand, imagining the breeze on my face and watching the waves hitting the sand.

Guided imagery is the process of being guided through calming or helpful mental images. This includes following along with a description of a peaceful place or calming scene, healing process, or other guided images. An example of guided imagery would be my saying to you:

Close your eyes, and now imagine you are lying on a white sandy beach.

A cold drink is in your right hand

You can hear the faint sounds of the waves crashing in the distance.

You feel a cool breeze pass over your body as you smell the salty sea air.

It's always best to perform visualization and guided imagery in a calm and relaxing environment. Trying to picture yourself on the beaches of Mexico while the dog is barking, phone is ringing, and kids are jumping on the couch—isn't the ideal situation to help you take a mental/visual vacation.

Chapter 8
How to Reduce Swelling

What is Swelling?

Swelling is an expansion of the volume of a part of the body due to a buildup of fluid. Organs, skin, or other body parts enlarge because of a buildup of fluid in the tissues. This is called edema. Swelling is the result of the increased movement of fluid and white blood cells into an area of inflammation. The release of chemicals and the compression of nerves in the area of injury cause pain. Pain and swelling are the body's natural warning mechanisms to protect it from further injury. However, often the body's response is excessive, and causes you too much pain and swelling.

What is Edema?

Edema is defined as excessive fluid buildup in tissues after the fluid leaks into the interstitial space. This means that fluid accumulates between the cells and the tiny blood vessels called capillaries, which leak fluid into the surrounding tissue. This results in swelling. Leaking capillaries cause your kidneys to accumulate higher than normal amounts of sodium (salt) and water to try to compensate for the capillary fluid loss. This results in more blood volume circulating in the body, which in turn causes even more capillary leakage into the surrounding tissue, which produces additional swelling—a vicious cycle. Lymphatic vessels pick up the fluid that leaks into your tissues from your bloodstream and return it to your circulatory system. Edema occurs when the lymphatic vessels get backed up or overloaded.

Edema may be a result of many things besides tissue trauma—including poor circulation, heart failure, blood clots, lymph node resection (removal) during cancer treatment, kidney failure, pregnancy, and liver disease. Other causes of edema include allergic reactions, sunburns, malnutrition, exposure to high altitude, and hormonal changes.

What is Postoperative Swelling?

As a physical therapist, I see patients all the time who have postoperative edema. This is swelling due to surgery or another injury causing tissue trauma. Even though surgery creates a controlled wound designed to make you better, inflammation and swelling are your body's natural reaction to surgery, and thus injury, and cannot be avoided. Too much swelling for a prolonged period of time can result in postoperative edema. This can constrict the affected body area and cause excessive pain. Too much swelling can restrict your range of motion and will also create problems with internal scarring. These issues can lengthen your overall recovery from the surgery.

What Makes Swelling Worse?

Physical Inactivity

Edema is more common among people who do not exercise at all, and walk very little. An inactive lifestyle will increase edema. Lymph circulation is positively affected, and moves, by muscle contraction.

My recommendation: keep moving to move that lymph fluid!

Positioning

Poor positioning of the affected area can cause that area to swell even more. Edema is affected by gravity, which makes the area that is in a dependent position swell more. For example, if you had liposuction of your thighs and you stand all day, chances are your lower legs will be more swollen because gravity causes the swelling to pool in your legs.

My recommendation: elevating the part of the body that is swollen will help reduce the swelling.

Large Amounts of Fat Removal

When fat is removed from the body, it leaves an empty space. The body recognizes this space and wants to correct the balance of the body, so it fills the area with fluid to maintain homeostasis. Therefore, the more fat that is removed, the more swelling you will have.

My recommendation: pay extra attention to doing swelling-reducing treatments after liposuction. I discuss it in detail in upcoming sections.

Heat

Heat causes your capillaries to widen, which leads to an increase in the leakage of fluid into tissues, thus adding to swelling and pain. Be aware that you will be more swollen on hot or humid days. For optimal healing, stay in a cool, dry environment, i.e. air conditioning in hot weather, for the first few weeks after surgery. Avoid hot tubs and saunas, and limit hot showers to less than 15 minutes at a time. Don't apply a heating pad to the swollen area.

My recommendation: don't book a trip to a hot or humid place shortly after surgery. I've had patients who have scheduled trips to the Caribbean a week after liposuction and then wonder why they look fatter than they did before surgery. It's not fat—it's increased swelling!

I also recommend patients schedule surgery in the cooler months. If you are having surgery in the middle of the summer when it is hot and humid, it will work less in your favor than if you scheduled it during the cooler fall/winter months.

Medication

Many medications can increase swelling, including vasodilators (drugs that open blood vessels); calcium channel blockers; NSAIDs (non-steroidal anti-inflammatory medications); contraceptive pills and estrogens; chemotherapy agents; some medications for diabetes mellitus such as pioglitazone and rosiglitazone; corticosteroids such as prednisone and methylprednisolone; and pramipexole. Also, prescription pain medications often cause increased swelling and/or bloating.

My recommendation: before your surgery, talk with your doctor about medications you are taking, or will be taking, that can cause more swelling.

Excessive Sodium Intake

Consumption of too much salt in combination with too much fluid will cause fluid retention. We heard me go on and on in the diet and nutrition chapter—but I'll say it again—salt causes swelling. Don't consume it.

My recommendation: during recovery, avoid salty foods such as soup, sushi and pickles. They are not your friends!

Malnutrition or Bad Diet

Dietitians say that low consumption of vitamin B1, as well as deficiencies in vitamins B6 and B5, may contribute toward fluid retention. Low protein levels could lead to increased swelling as well.

My recommendation: be sure you are eating a healthy balanced diet and taking a multivitamin, well before your surgery.

Scar Tissue

Scar tissue increases swelling and edema because it blocks lymphatic flow, so fluid gets stuck in the area.

My recommendation: work on minimizing scar tissue, as discussed in the upcoming chapters.

Menstrual Cycle

Hormone levels fluctuate during the menstrual cycle. During the week just before menstrual bleeding, the reduction in the levels of the hormone progesterone may cause fluid retention.

My recommendation: attempt to schedule your surgery date just after your period, and not the week of. Since this might not always be possible, be aware of the effect your menstrual cycle will have on swelling. Also be aware that surgery may disrupt your menstrual cycle schedule, causing it to come early or be delayed.

Menopause

Around the time of menopause, as well as after it, hormone fluctuations can cause fluid retention. Hormone replacement therapy after menopause can also cause edema.

My recommendation: be aware that hormone replacement therapies can cause more swelling and affect your recovery period. Tell your surgeon about any hormone replacement treatments you are taking.

Genetics

We often underestimate the role of genetics in how our bodies respond. Genetics play a huge part in many things, including postoperative swelling.

My recommendation: there is nothing you can do about genetics. Just deal with it and hope your genetics work in your favor.

Skin Type

Certain skin types tend to retain more fluid than others. It is my observation that those with olive complexions—people of Mediterranean or Indian descent—tend to have more swelling. People with thicker skin are more prone to increased swelling.

My recommendation: if your skin type puts you at higher risk for swelling, you need to pay special attention to the rest of this chapter, and to Chapters 9 and 10.

High Altitudes

Especially when combined with physical exertion, being at a high altitude, even for a short period of time, can cause fluid retention.

My recommendation: don't take an airplane trip soon after your surgery.

Poor Skin Care

Poor skin care can cause skin breakdown and cause poor healing.

My recommendation: cleanse your skin with hypoallergenic soap, moisturize with perfume-free lotion, and make sure you follow the section on proper skin and incision care for the area affected by your surgery, as recommended by your doctor.

What is a Seroma?

A seroma is a pool of fluid that develops in tissue after surgery. It usually develops in the stomach area, most often the lower stomach. You can tell you have a seroma because when you touch it, you see a "waterbed effect." You can see the fluid underneath moving in a wavelike pattern. It is not dangerous but can lead to an infection. What causes a seroma? It happens for different reasons. It can happen when large amounts of fat are removed at once, failure to drain after surgery, the patient is eating a high sodium diet, certain medications, scar tissue around the area, and genetics. It is difficult to get rid of and will often have to be treated by the doctor removing the fluid with a needle. The best way to prevent a seroma is eat a low sodium diet, wear your compression garment and discuss any medications you are taking with your doctor.

Treatment of Postoperative Swelling

You can take steps to minimize postoperative swelling and edema. Although I gave some suggestions above, you may be wondering: what else you can do.

While I was training to become a physical therapist, I learned that the gold standard for treatment of swelling is something called RICE, which stands for rest, ice, compression, and elevation.

This basic principle of healing is something that my profession carries over to treat many different medical issues. The RICE principle, combined with skin care and other techniques, is discussed in this chapter and the remaining chapters of this book. So let me help guide you during your recovery phase!

Rest

Rest refers to your need to limit your activity so your wound does not undergo unnecessary trauma. But rest is relative. What I mean is that you should move the affected area gently to keep it mobile and prevent stiffness during healing but not so much that you increase the pain and swelling. It is very good to rest and recuperate on your couch, but that doesn't mean you should lay there like a mummy—movement is necessary! You should keep moving the affected area gently at times during the first few days. Movement promotes the pumping of blood and limits stiffness. You can keep all non-affected areas moving. Regular exercise helps improve lymph drainage. However, in some people, strenuous exercise can cause or worsen swelling. See the following parts of this chapter for exercise that can be done to promote healing.

Ice

Ice, ice, baby! Ice is so important. To reduce the normal side effects of going under the knife, using ice regularly is important. The goal is to limit fluid accumulation in the injured area by reducing blood flow to the area—and ice does just that! Cold temperatures reduce blood flow to the affected area, thus decreasing swelling or bleeding in the tissue. Using ice is key in reducing swelling! Think of your body like a sprained ankle—the more ice right after the "injury," the better. Ice helps keep the swelling down!

Use caution when using ice

Typically, doctors will prescribe pain medication after surgery, but one side effect of pain medication can be skin numbness. If your skin is numb, you are more prone to frostbite. So icing your wound could be potentially dangerous unless you pay attention to how you are doing it. Here are some tips to make sure that you are icing your injury effectively and safely:

- Apply ice for the first 72 hours, 20–30 minutes on and 30 minutes off—leaving the ice on longer actually reverses its effect, and may increase swelling.
- Do not use heat for the first 72 hours as heat will increase the swelling.
- Chemical ice packs should never be applied directly to the skin because frostbite can occur.
- To ice large areas, i.e. abdomen or entire thigh, the best method is to fill a small plastic garbage bag with cubed or crushed ice. You may want to double-bag it so it does not leak or get too cold.

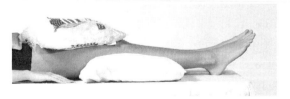

Photo 1: Using a bag of ice on a large area, here on a thigh

Traditional ice packs are okay, but do not conform well to the contours of the body, so they are not the most efficient of choices.

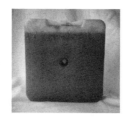

Photo 2: A traditional ice pack

There are many different types of ice therapy products on the market. It is up you to determine what works best for you.

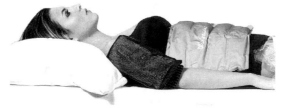

Photo 3: An example of a contoured ice pack for the stomach and arm

For a smaller area that require contour, i.e. the eyes or nose, a bag of frozen peas works great.

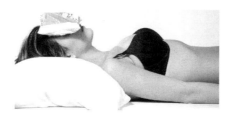

Photo 4: A package of frozen peas makes a flexible ice pack for the face

Aqueduct Medical, Inc. makes new and interesting body-conforming cooling packs, specifically designed for post-cosmetic surgery.

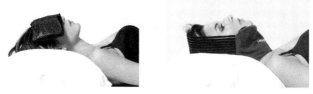

Photo 5A-B: Two examples of contoured ice packs available for use after cosmetic surgery

Skin Care

Apply fragrance-free moisturizer, each day, to prevent chapped skin. Avoid cuts, burns, needle sticks, or other injury to the affected area. If you shave, use an electric razor to reduce the chance of cutting the skin.

Avoid sun exposure on the operated area for one year. When you are outside, wear a broad-spectrum sunscreen that protects against both UVA and UVB radiation and has a sun protection factor (SPF) of at least 30.

Sun, heat, and humidity negatively affect swelling. They will make you seriously swell and bloat! Stay out of the sun for at least a month after surgery. Trust me on this! For those people who schedule their liposuction surgery on May 15th and think they will be beach ready for Labor Day—you are seriously wrong. You will be a swollen puff if you bask in the sun two weeks after surgery. Give yourself at least two months before being beach ready after most procedures.

I have had so many patients who schedule trips in tropical places to "recover after surgery." Huge mistake! This will just make recovery harder. If you don't believe me, try it, and you will literally see yourself bloating right before your eyes!

Compression

Compression is so important that it gets a chapter to itself. Chapter 9 is devoted to a discussion of garments and compression, after an introduction to compression and lymphatic drainage massage at the end of this chapter.

Elevation and Positioning

While resting after surgery, positioning can affect swelling and therefore affect healing.

For the first 24–48 hours after your procedure, the affected body part should be elevated as much as you can. While resting, try and change your position about every 30 minutes.

Try to keep your operative area above the level of your heart. This does not apply to the abdomen. As for the abdomen, swelling that moves from side to side is usually affected by which part is in contact with the bed, i.e. in a gravity-dependent position. So, if you lie on one side more than the other, the side you lie on the most will usually be more swollen.

1. Positioning after Abdominal Surgery

Sleeping on your stomach is discouraged for the first couple weeks. In Stage 1, begin by sleeping flat with your legs slightly bent—you can achieve this by placing pillows under your knees. In Stage 2, after several days when you are able to more comfortably move around, you may feel comfortable sleeping on your side. Placing a pillow between your knees may provide additional comfort when you are sleeping on your side. If you choose to sleep on your side, make sure to rotate between sleeping on your left and right side—if you do not rotate sides, swelling will pool in the side of your abdomen that you sleep on the most. In Stage 3, after 7 to 10 days, try to lie flat to prevent swelling from pooling in your midsection.

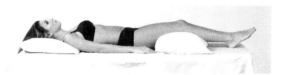

Photo 6: Sleeping flat with your legs slightly bent (pillow under knees) immediately after abdominal surgery (Stage 1).

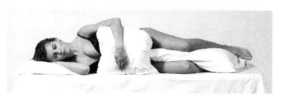

Photo 7: Using a pillow between knees for comfort while sleeping on your side (Stage 2).

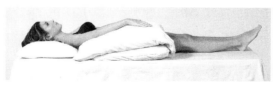

Photo 8: Progress to sleeping flat to prevent midsection swelling (Stage 3).

2. Positioning after Arm Surgery

Prop your arms up when lying, sitting, and relaxing. Use extra pillows for sleeping and try to keep your hand and arm above the level of your heart. Resting with the affected area above your heart level will encourage swelling to return towards your torso instead of collecting in your arms and hands. Swelling is hard to get rid of after it pools in the hand and lower arm.

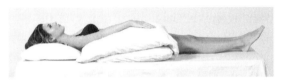

Photo 9: Proper resting position of arm and hand after surgery (elevated above the heart).

3. Positioning after Buttock Surgery

Do not lie on your back—sleeping on your stomach is the preferred position. If lying flat on your stomach is difficult, placing a pillow under your abdomen may increase your comfort, and a bigger pillow may provide more comfort than a smaller pillow. Check with your doctor to determine if it's okay for you to sleep on your side.

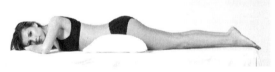

Photo 10:A Sleeping position after buttock surgery with pillow under pelvis.

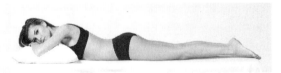

Photo 10B: Sleeping position after buttock surgery
Option B is on stomach with no pillow under pelvis.

4. Positioning after Breast or Pectoral Surgery

Sleeping with your head elevated above heart level will allow gravity to prevent swelling from pooling in your chest. If your doctor allows you to sleep on your side instead of your back, maintain elevation of your head. Make sure to rotate sleeping between your left and right side so swelling will not pool in the side you sleep on the most. Do not sleep on your stomach. Your doctor will let you know when it is okay to start lying on your stomach.

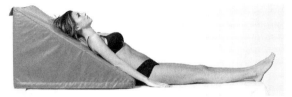

Photo 11A: Sleeping position after breast or pectoral surgery—upper body elevated.

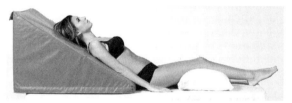

Photo 11B: Modify the position by placing a pillow under your knees for comfort.

5. Positioning after Calf, Leg, or Thigh Surgery

Prop your legs up when relaxing in a lying or sitting position. Use extra pillows for sleeping and try to keep your legs above the level of your heart. Resting with the affected area above heart level will encourage swelling to return towards your torso instead of collecting in your legs and feet. When swelling collects in your lower legs and feet, it is hard to get rid of because your feet are in a dependent position when standing and walking.

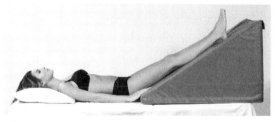

Photo 12: Resting position after leg, calf, or thigh surgery

6. Positioning after Facial, Head, Neck, Nose, or Ear Surgery

Sleeping with your head elevated above heart level will allow gravity to move the swelling down and out of your head, neck, and face. If you choose to sleep on your side instead of your back—but don't sleep on your side after ear surgery—maintain elevation of your head. Make sure to alternate sleeping on your left and right side, or else swelling will pool in the side of your face you sleep on the most. Do not sleep on your stomach.

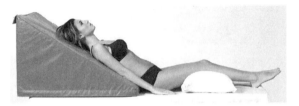

Photo 13: Resting position after facial, head, neck, nose or ear surgery.

Exercises to Reduce Swelling

Decongestive exercises are gentle and move fluid out of the affected area. Unlike the cardiovascular system which has the heart, the lymphatic system does not have an active pump to propel lymphatic fluid back to the bloodstream. Effective lymph flow depends on muscle and joint activity. The exercises in this section are intended for Stage 1 of your recovery. The purpose of the decongestive exercises is to decrease swelling and increase range of motion in the affected areas. Decongestive exercises are most effective when performed while the patient wears compression garments or bandages. For best results, decongestive exercise protocols are performed two to three times a day for the first month after surgery. Following the exercises, the patient should rest with the affected limb elevated for at least ten minutes. Always check with your doctor before beginning any exercise program. Stop any exercise if you experience pain.

General Exercises after Any Surgery

The following five exercises are typically safe to be performed after all types of surgery. These exercises are intended to increase blood flow and circulation.

1. Elevated ankle pumps

Lie on your back with your foot elevated on a couple of pillows.

Move foot up and down, pumping the ankle.

Perform two sets of 20 repetitions twice a day.

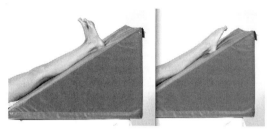

Photo 14A-B: Elevated ankle pumps

2. Heel slides

Lie on your back with legs straight.

Slide heel along floor toward buttock.

Return to original position and repeat.

Perform two sets of 10 repetitions, twice a day.

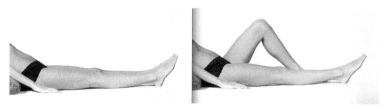

Photo 15A-B: Heel slides

3. Knee extension

Also known as long arc quadriceps stretch (LAQS).

Sitting with your feet flat on floor and your back in neutral position, straighten knee.

Return to original position and repeat.

Perform two sets of 10 repetitions twice a day.

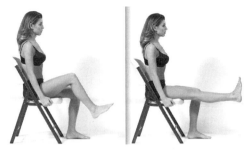

Photo 16A-B: Knee extensions (LAQS)

4. Seated marches

Sitting with your feet flat on floor, gently march in place.
Perform two sets of 10 repetitions twice a day.

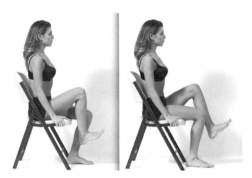

Photo 17A-B: Seated marches

5. Shoulder rolls

Stand or sit.

Raise your shoulders towards ears and roll backwards.

Return to start position.

Perform two sets of 10 repetitions, twice a day.

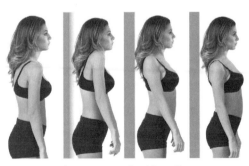

Photo 18A-D: Shoulder rolls

Exercise after Abdominal Surgery

Abdominal breathing

This basic exercise is typically safe and can be performed after any procedure on the abdomen, i.e. abdominoplasty, body lift, or liposuction. The purpose of this exercise is to decrease swelling and decongest the area by contracting the diaphragm.

Begin by placing both hands flat on your belly, over your diaphragm.

Inhale slowly.

Breathe deeply through your nose, allowing your stomach to expand into your hand (8 seconds).

As air enters your lungs, your stomach should expand outwards, not the chest.

Breathe out slowly through pursed lips, allowing your stomach to flatten (8 seconds).

Repeat five times, with a short rest between each breath to avoid dizziness.

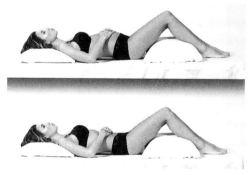

Photo 19A-B: Abdominal breathing

Exercises after Arm Surgery

The following eight exercises are basic and typically safe to be performed after any procedure on the upper arm, i.e. liposuction or arm lift. The purpose of these exercises is to decrease swelling and decongest the upper extremity.

1. Elevated hand pumps

Elevate your arms on a few pillows, so they are above your heart level.

Begin with your fingers straight and spread apart.

Close your hands into a fist.

Open and spread fingers. Repeat.

Perform two sets of 20 repetitions twice a day.

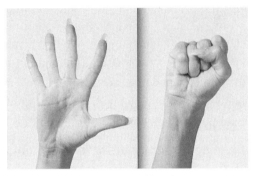

Photo 20A-B: Elevated hand pumps

2. Hand pump with squeeze ball

Lie with your arms elevated on a couple of pillows, above heart level.

Place ball in your palm.

Close your hand and squeeze ball.

Perform two sets of 20 repetitions twice a day.

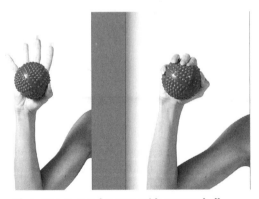

Photo 21A-B: Hand pumps with squeeze ball

3. Arm raises

Lie on your back with your arms at your side, palms facing in.
Move one arm over your head, with elbows straight.
Return to start position and repeat.
Perform two sets of 10 repetitions twice a day.

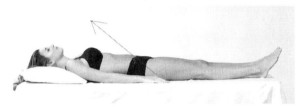

Photo 22: Arm raises

4. Elbow flexion and extension

Sit or lie with your arms elevated on a pillow.
Begin with your arms straight, palms up.
Bend your elbow upward.
Return to starting position.
Perform two sets of 10 repetitions twice a day.

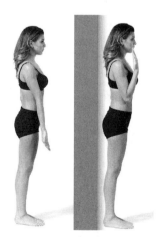

Photo 23A-B: Elbow flexion and extension

5. Triceps extension

Stand, leaning over a chair or table.

Start with your elbow bent and straighten elbow through available range.

Return to start position.

Perform two sets of 10 repetitions twice a day.

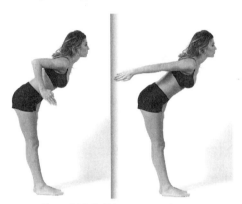

Photo 24A-B: Triceps extension

6. Shoulder rolls

Stand or sit. Raise your shoulders towards your ears.

Roll shoulders backwards.

Return to start position.

Perform two sets of 20 repetitions twice a day.

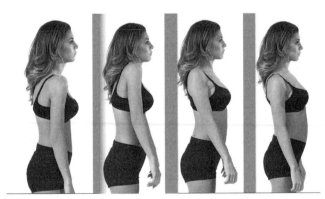

Photo 25A-D: Shoulder rolls

7. Arm raises to the side (abduction)

Stand or sit with your arms at your sides, palms forward.

Lift your arms out and above your head.

Keep your elbows straight.

Return to start position and repeat.

Perform two sets of 10 repetitions twice a day.

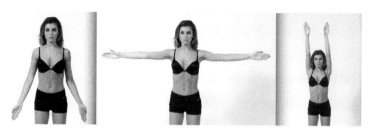

Photo 26A-C: Arm raises to the side

8. Arm circles

Stand or sit with your arms straight out to sides, palms out.

Make circles with your outstretched arms, keeping your elbows straight.

Return to start position and repeat.

Perform two sets of 10 repetitions twice a day.

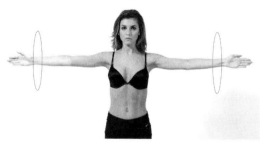

Photo 27: Arm circles

Exercise after Back or Flank Surgery

The following exercise is typically safe to be performed after back or flank surgery. The purpose of this exercise is to decrease swelling and decongest the area.

Cat and Camel exercise

Position yourself on your hands and knees.

Gently lower your back down, forming an arch.

Then gently raise your back up towards the ceiling, creating a hump.

Perform two sets of 10 repetitions twice a day.

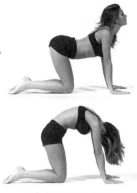

Photo 28A-B: Cat and Camel exercise

Exercise after Buttock Surgery

The following basic exercise, called glut sets, is typically safe to be performed after buttock lift or buttock augmentation surgery. The purpose of this exercise is to decrease swelling and decongest the area.

Glut sets

Lie on your stomach with your legs extended.

Squeeze your buttocks together and then release. Repeat.

Perform two sets of 10 repetitions twice a day.

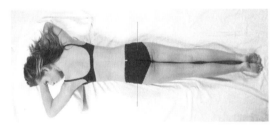

Photo 29: Glut sets

Exercises after Facial Surgery

The following six basic exercises are typically safe and are to be performed after any procedure on the face, i.e. rhinoplasty, brow lift, or chin augmentation. The purpose of these exercises is to decrease swelling and decongest the area.

1. Forehead elevation and depression

Frown your eyebrows to midline, and then raise them. Repeat.
Perform two sets of 10 repetitions, twice a day.

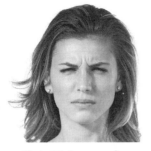 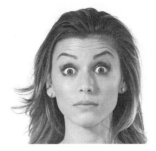

Photo 30: Frown eyebrows   Photo 31: Raise eyebrows

2. Eye closing and opening

Squeeze your eyes tightly closed, and then open widely. Repeat.
Perform two sets of 10 repetitions twice a day.

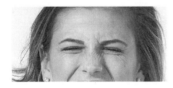 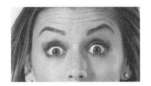

Photo 32: Eye closing   Photo 33: Eye opening

3. Cheek raises

Lift your cheeks upward, causing wrinkles in your nose. Then make an expression of distaste.
Perform two sets of 10 repetitions twice a day.

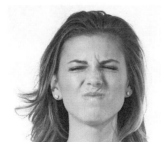 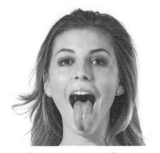

Photo 34: Wrinkle Nose   Photo 35: Express distaste

4. Neck tightening

Draw the corners of your mouth downward.

Tighten muscles on neck to tighten the skin below the jaw.

Perform two sets of 10 repetitions twice a day.

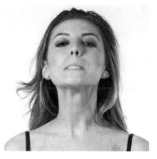

Photo 36: Neck tightening

5. Smile and lip purse

Raise sides of your mouth and make a big smile.

Then purse your lips together as if sucking through a straw.

Perform two sets of 10 repetitions twice a day.

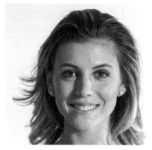

Photo 37: Big smile

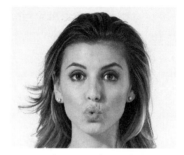

Photo 38: Lip pursing

6. Cheek puffing

Puff your cheeks out, filling them up with air.

Allow them to deflate and repeat.

Perform two sets of 10 repetitions twice a day.

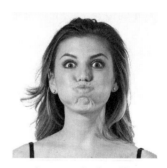

Photo 39: Cheek puffing

Exercises after Leg Surgery

The following eight basic exercises are typically safe and are to be performed after any procedure on the thigh and calf, i.e. liposuction, thigh lift, or calf augmentation. The purpose of these exercises is to decrease swelling and decongest the lower extremity.

1. Elevated ankle pumps

Lie on your back with your foot elevated on a couple of pillows.
Move foot up and down, pumping the ankle.
Perform two sets of 20 repetitions twice a day.

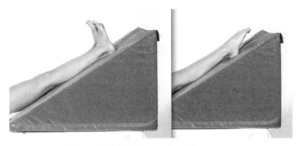

Photo 40A-B: Elevated ankle pumps

2. Ankle alphabet

Lie on your back with your foot elevated on a couple of pillows.
Slowly draw the letters of the alphabet, leading with your big toe.
Do not move your hip or knee.
Perform one set twice a day.

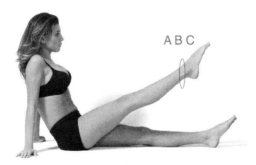

Photo 41: Ankle alphabet

3. Quad sets

Sit with your leg extended.

Tighten your knee, trying to push the knee into the floor.

Hold for 10 seconds, and then release your knee. Repeat.

Perform two sets of 10 repetitions twice a day.

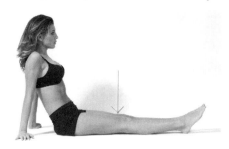

Photo 42: Quad sets

4. Heel slides

Lie on your back with legs straight.

Slide heel along floor toward your buttock.

Return to original position and repeat.

Perform two sets of 10 repetitions, twice a day.

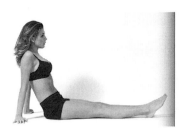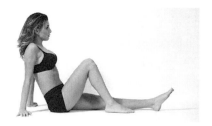

Photo 43A-B: Heel slides

5. Hip abduction

Lie on your back, with your legs straight and together.

Move one leg out to the side, keeping your knee straight.

Make sure your toes and knee are always facing forward, not rolling out to the side.

Perform two sets of 10 repetitions twice a day.

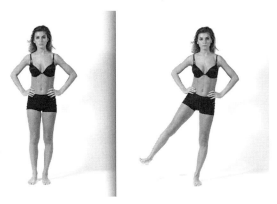

Photo 44A-B: Hip abduction

6. Knee extension

Also called short arc quadriceps stretch (SAQS)

Lie on your back with a pillow under your knee.

Bend your knee to 45 degrees.

Straighten your leg, tightening the knee.

Return to original position and repeat.

Perform two sets of 10 repetitions twice a day.

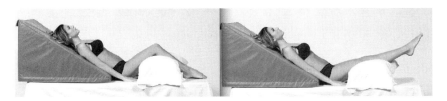

Photo 45A-B: Knee extension (SAQS)

7. Knee extension (LAQS)

Also known as long arc quadriceps stretch (LAQS)

Sit with your feet flat on floor and your back in neutral position.

Straighten your knee.

Return to original position and repeat.

Perform two sets of 10 repetitions, twice a day.

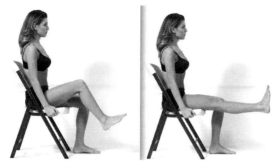

Photo 46A-B: Knee extension (LAQS)

8. Hamstring curl on stomach

Lie face down with your legs straight.

Bend your knee, bringing your heel towards your buttock.

Return to start position. Do not let buttocks or hips rise upward.

Perform two sets of 10 repetitions twice a day.

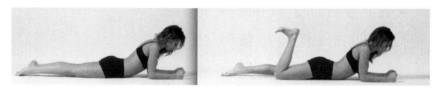

Photo 47A-B: Hamstring curl on stomach

Compression

Compression garments are specially designed elastic apparel worn after surgical procedures and throughout recovery. They provide additional support by contouring to the body or body part to improve blood circulation, minimize swelling after the procedure, flush the body out of potentially harmful fluids, accelerate the healing process, and allow the patient to return to daily routines sooner. A compression garment also provides support to surgical areas for more comfort and helps the skin fit better to its new contours.

Plastic surgeons generally recommend use of compression garments following tummy tucks, liposuction, arm lifts, facelifts, facial procedures, gastric bypass procedures, male mastopexy, breast augmentation, breast reduction, and many other types of surgical sculpture procedures. Not all surgeons will recommend compression garments, traditionally those who come from an old-fashioned school of thought. My observations have determined garments are essential for optimal healing.

A compression garment worn after any procedure needs to be a specific type of medical garment that has the proper amount of compression pressure—the amount of compression should not be so much that blood supply is cut off or pain is increased. Using a garment that is not a medically specified garment may create a problem for you and your recovery. Typically, compression garments are used in two stages. Stage 1 garments are used for the first month after surgery and Stage 2 garments are used starting two months after surgery.

See Chapter 9 for step-by-step instructions on proper compression for healing.

Lymphatic Drainage Massage

Lymphatic drainage massage (LDM) is a manual technique used by physical therapists to reduce edema. It involves very gentle massage techniques in specific areas of the body in a particular order to stimulate lymph drainage. It is particularly effective for edema control. Massage combined with compression is one of the most effective treatment strategies for postoperative swelling and edema.

See Chapter 10 for detailed instructions on LDM treatment.

Chapter 9

Compression Garments
Reduce Swelling

Wearing a compression garment after cosmetic surgery is essential for healing! This is a staple for healing in the "Psomas Method." Compression aims to decrease the swelling that results from the inflammatory process after cosmetic surgery. Even though swelling after surgery is going to happen no matter what, too much swelling results in loss of function, excessive pain, eventual slowing of blood flow due to blood vessel restriction, and slower results.

A medical compression garment can be one of the most important factors in improving the results of your healing process. Other factors, i.e. how the garment fits and how often you wear it, can also greatly affect your outcome.

Compression garments should always be used after liposuction surgery. Other types of surgery after which compression garments are commonly used are after tummy tuck, body lifts, and breast or buttock implants. Bandaging is used after most facial surgeries and often do not require an actual garment.

Typically, if you are required to wear a garment after surgery your surgeon will prescribe it for you, but some doctors are still not recommending them. *It is your choice which recommendation to follow, but in my over 10 years of expertise in this area, believe me compression garments work.* Some doctors will require that a patient purchase a garment prior to surgery and bring it with them on surgery day. Other surgeons will have a supply of medical compression garments available and will fit the patient immediately after the surgery is completed. It is very difficult for patients to determine on their own what a suitable garment is. It is strongly recommended that a patient be measured and fitted by a garment specialist at a medical supply store. Always consult with your doctor before beginning to wear a compression garment.

Why is a Compression Garment Necessary?

A compression garment is needed postoperatively to decrease swelling and help you heal smoothly and evenly. Period. You need it—no debates. Some doctors have really laid-back attitudes on wearing a compression garment. You can take their word for it and see how you do. My patients look like a million bucks and wearing a compression garment is one of the staples of their recovery process.

If you don't want to take my word for it, here is the science behind it. During cosmetic surgery procedures, inflammation occurs when underlying tissue—fat, blood vessels, and lymphatic system—is traumatized as expected, causing leakage of fluid and blood into tissue. During certain procedures, i.e. liposuction, large amounts of fat are removed, leaving an empty space where the fat once was. Because the human body will not allow that space to remain vacant, that new space fills up with fluid to maintain balance.

Your body is largely made up of water, and thus your body needs to balance the amounts of liquid between your cells, and in your blood. If too much fluid stays between the cells, too little returns to the blood. This causes your heart to pump much harder and your body to swell. Swelling creates problems that slow down your healing during recovery from surgery. Swelling interferes with smooth and even healing of your body. Also, it prevents your skin from firmly re-adhering to your body. When fluid accumulates, it can prevent oxygen and nutrients from reaching the area, which also can impact healing. In rare cases, if healing is severely impacted, excessive swelling can cause some cells to die. Infection is another possible side effect of poor healing. If those pooled fluids progress into the serious complication called a blood clot, you could die. A compression garment pushes down on the skin and squeezes body fluids back toward deeper tissues, reducing the swelling in the affected areas. An extra advantage of surgical compression garments is that loose skin is held firmly against the body, allowing the connective tissue to tightly and normally re-adhere during healing.

Non-Compliance with Wearing Your Garment

Studies show that patients who do not wear a garment do not heal as fast. Non-compliant patients have greater amounts of swelling than patients who wear a garment.

If you don't wear an appropriate garment as directed, you are at greater risk for:

1. Pockets of swelling which go on to form uneven and lumpy areas.
2. Fluid build-up that may stretch your skin and cause improper reattachment of your skin to your body's new contours. This means the skin does not heal as flat and taut.
3. Swelling that can cause tape, sutures, staples, or other fastenings that close a surgical site to break or dislocate. Then your wound can break open and gape.

Ill-fitting or poorly designed compression garments:

1. Increase risk of seroma, a pocket of clear fluid that sometimes develops in the body after surgery.
2. May cause lymphedema, the accumulation of lymph fluid in the soft tissue that causes swelling, often of your arms and legs. This is sometimes worsened by inflammation, obstruction, or removal of lymph channels.
3. Can cause lumpy or uneven skin.
4. Can irritate incisions and cause exaggerated and/or red scars.
5. Can cause necrosis (death) of skin and other tissues.
6. May cut off vital blood circulation to the surgical site.

What is the Right Compression Garment?

Correct compression garments reduce fluid build-up, promote steady flow of fluid, increase blood circulation, promote proper skin adhesion to newly contoured areas, reduce side effects of surgery, reduce risk of infection, and hold surgical dressings in place until they are ready to be removed.

The five characteristics of a proper post-surgical medical garment are proper fit, design, fabric type and tension, amount of pressure, and wearing schedule.

Fit

An improperly fitting compression garment can do more harm than good. The compression garment should stay in place and not fold or form rolls. While you may like your clothes to be a little too big and to fold because you've lost weight, a compression garment that is too big and folds or rolls can cut off circulation or exert too much pressure underneath the fold or roll. I recommend getting a garment with shoulder straps to prevent folding and to help the garment stay in place.

Fitting rule #1

The garment should cross the joint above and below the area that was operated on. The most important factor in the fit of a garment is making sure the garment is longer, higher, and covers a larger area than the operated area.

Example 1

If you had liposuction of the abdomen, the garment should start right under the breast, cover the entire abdomen, and go below the hipbone. If your garment cuts in at the navel, it will create increased swelling in the upper abdomen—a muffin top! You could potentially have a worse shape than you did before surgery.

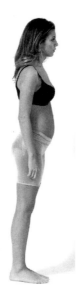
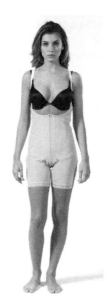

Photo 1: Wrong fit of garment after liposuction of the abdomen

Photo 2: Right fit of garment after liposuction of the abdomen

Example 2

After liposuction of the thighs, if you wear a garment that stops mid-thigh or above the knee, swelling will accumulate at the knee. The garment must go to the knee joint or past the knee joint.

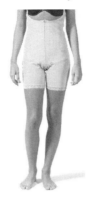 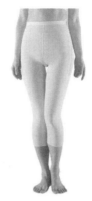

Photo 3: Wrong fit of garment after liposuction of the thighs   *Photo 4: Right fit of garment after liposuction of the thighs*

Fitting rule #2

If you had surgery on more than one area, the garment must take into account all areas of surgery.

Example

If you had liposuction of the abdomen and the thighs, the garment cannot just take care of the thighs—it must cover the entire abdomen as well as your thighs. The same garment that was right in the previous scenario is wrong in this scenario!

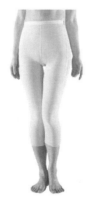 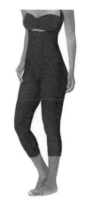

Photo 5: Wrong fit of garment after liposuction of abdomen and thighs   *Photo 6: Right fit of garment after liposuction of abdomen and thighs*

Fitting rule #3

Swelling will always pool further away from the area of compression, so it is important to cover the whole area.

Example

After liposuction of the upper arm, if you have a tight garment that goes to the top of the elbow, you may get swelling in the forearm. The way to combat this is to make sure the garment goes to the forearm.

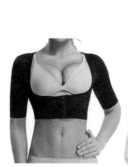

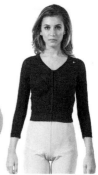

Photo 7: Wrong fit of garment after liposuction of arms

Photo 8: Right fit of garment after liposuction of arms

Fitting rule #4

When an area is compressed with a garment, swelling will accumulate in any open area.

Example 1

In this picture of a hand wearing a compression bandage, you can see an opening in the middle and a small opening on the side. These open areas will get very swollen because they are not covered by the garment. The swelling gets forced out into the open space.

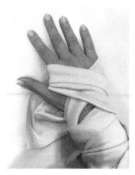

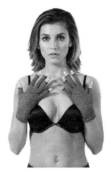

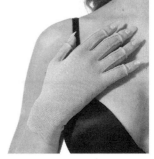

Photo 9: Wrong fit of compression of hand

Photo 10A-B: Right fit of compression of

Example 2

Most compression garments for the torso come with an opening in the genital area, so you can urinate. What the garment companies have not taken into consideration is that opening causes swelling to pool there because of fitting rule #4.

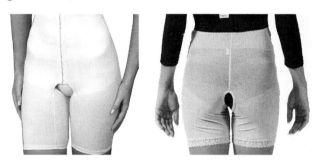

Photo 11A-B: Examples of opening at genital area where swelling can accumulate

After I had my surgery, I woke up one morning and went to use the bathroom—I almost freaked out! My vaginal area was so swollen it was hanging out of the opening of the garment. Um, ew. I thought I was having an allergic reaction, but then my physical therapist brain kicked in and I realized what was happening. I knew this was because there was an opening in the garment and the swelling rushes to the area where there is no compression. I had to add compression in this area or it would stay swollen. So, I stuck a maxi pad in the hole. Viola! Problem solved. By the next morning my lady part was back to normal.

Tip!

I advise my patients to fix the problem by placing a thick, disposable maxi pad in the open area. This will add the compression you need.

Fitting rule #5

Uneven compression—areas of tightness and looseness—will cause bad results.

Example

Look at the first picture. The Ace wrapping is uneven, tighter in the middle, and the pressure is not consistent throughout. The circular technique of the wrapping will cause a tourniquet effect. This will interfere with giving the arm a smooth, even appearance. The bandaging should be flat and even.

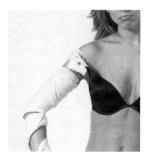 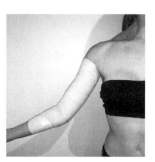

Photo 12: Uneven bandaging of the arm

Photo 13: Even bandaging of the arm

Design

A quality compression garment is designed with features to ensure comfort. This could include:

Seamless panels at surgical incision sites

Flat seams

Consistent pressure

Anatomically correct open groin area, with or without a flap

Run-resistant fabric

Accurate support to specific areas of the body

Fabric Type and Tension

It is important to use a certified medical compression garment. The ideal material is a woven Lycra-Spandex mix. The fabric and its composition are essential when determining a product's purpose and delivering accurate compression or support. The fabric should provide constant and consistent compression. Many fabrics or weaves lose their compression properties or "memory" over time.

Amount of Pressure

The correct amount of pressure for a post-surgical garment can range from 15 to 40 mmHG (millimeters of mercury). Ideally it should be 25 to 35 mmHG. The greater the mmHG, the greater the compression.

A quality compression garment will apply constant and consistent pressure from all angles, for a long time, to provide support to the entire surgical region. The amount of pressure that the garment provides is one of the most important factors in healing. While compression garments are super helpful, too much compression can prolong swelling. Excessive compression, after all drainage has ceased, can impair the normal function of your capillaries. On the flip side, too little compression will allow swelling within the body.

One of my patients, Tom, took the liberty of wearing his own compression garment. He thought that bike shorts would be more comfortable—and a better fit—than a medical compression garment. But due to the wrong type of pressure as well as the inconsistent pressure that this type of fabric creates, fluid became trapped in his inner thigh. That fluid turned into lymphedema. It took months for him to recover from this mistake. You can read about his case in the last chapter.

I cannot stress enough to you how important correct compression garments are to your healing process!

Wearing Schedule

Generally, for good results, it is recommended that a garment be worn at least 23 hours a day for at least four to six weeks. If you can tolerate wearing the garment for six months up to one year, this will provide the best results. Mild discomfort is natural when wearing a garment, but research shows that patients who are 100 percent compliant with wearing their garment have greater satisfaction in the results of their procedure compared to patients who wear it less or do not wear it at all. So push through the discomfort because it will be worth it in the long run! It's a cliché but it's true—no pain, no gain!

Here is a list of typical minimum amounts of time a compression garment should be worn after a specific procedure:

Abdominoplasty .... At least 4-6 weeks

Breast augmentation .... At least 2 weeks

Breast reduction .... At least 6 weeks

Facelift .... At least 2 weeks

Liposuction .... At least 4-6 weeks

Lower body lift .... At least 4-6 weeks

Thigh or buttock lift .... At least 4-6 weeks

Upper arm lift .... At least 4-6 weeks

After my liposuction procedure I wore my phase one garment for eight weeks. Then I transitioned into my phase 2 Spanx® garment. I wore the Spanx® for a year. If I can do it, you can do it. The longer you wear the garments, the better.

Stage 1 versus Stage 2 Compression Garments

Common brands of medical compression garments are:

Annette	*Isavela*
ClearPoint Medical	*Make Me Heal*
Contemporary Design	*Marena*
DCL	*Rainey Compression Wear*
Design Veronique	*Solidea*

Stage 1 Garments

First-stage compression garments are worn immediately after surgery. Fluid needs to be expelled from of the area—this is where the open drainage process comes in. The use of postoperative compression garments during this stage is highly effective.

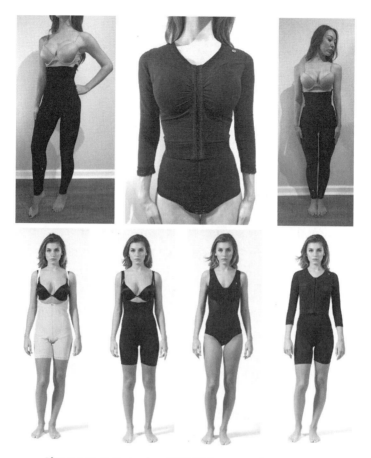

Photos 14A-G: Examples of STAGE 1 compression garments

Stage 2 Garments

Second-stage compression garments are worn after the initial Stage One medical garment. Most people transition into the second-stage garment after about four to six weeks.

Shapewear is commonly used as a Stage Two garment. But be careful! You must choose the right shapewear or you will do more harm than good.

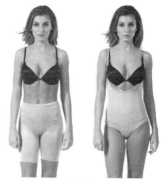

Photo 15A-B: Examples of Stage 2 garment

Remember the rules for garments

You want even compression, so don't choose shapewear with panels. Panels will cause pocket swelling.

Make sure the garment is long enough, high enough, and crosses two joints.

Make sure the fabric is strong enough—at least 15–20 mmHg but ideally 25–35 mmHg.

I love Spanx® shapewear. I think they are a great choice for Stage 2 because they are seamless, comfortable, and lightweight—and they do the job. In the many years I have worked as a physical therapist, I learned a very important lesson: if the homework I give my patients is too hard or too uncomfortable, they won't do it. I recommend Spanx® because most of my patients are compliant with wearing Spanx®. I can yell at them all day to wear their medical garments, but sometimes the garments are just too uncomfortable or too heavy to wear under certain outfits. Remember the rules when choosing the specific Spanx® style!

A good example of a Stage 2 garment is Spanx® Simplicity® Open Bust Mid-thigh. This is one of my favorite Spanx® pieces. I recommend it for Stage 2 use after abdominal or back liposuction. The reason I like it is because it goes both mid-thigh and high up on top. Also, it is made of a thicker, stronger material with even compression and no panels.

An example of a Stage 2 garment that I do not recommend is Spanx® Skinny Britches® Open Bust Mid-thigh. I do not recommend this version of the bodysuit after liposuction because of the paneling. The paneling will cause inconsistent pressure. It will put more pressure where the panels are and less pressure where the rest of the material is, so swelling will pool in the back and in the pockets of the crisscross.

Trust me—you will have better results and look better if you wear a correct medical compression garment.

Chapter 10
Using Massage to Reduce Swelling

History of Massage

Massage is an ancient therapy that dates back thousands of years. References to massage appear in literature from China, Japan, Greece, Rome, India, Egypt, and Arabic nations. In the 1850s massage techniques were brought from Sweden to the United States. They have been found to promote overall health and physical wellbeing, but the most commonly known purpose is the relaxation of muscles, which gives flexibility to tendons, tissues, and ligaments supporting better movement.

Purpose of Massage

As a physical therapist I have used massage techniques to ease the recovery of my patients for many different purposes. This is because the benefits of massage go way beyond muscle relaxation. There are numerous theories about how massage therapy can affect the body during the different stages of healing.

The gate control theory of pain suggests that massage may provide stimulation that helps to block pain signals sent to the brain. Other theories suggest that massage might stimulate the release of certain chemicals in the body, such as serotonin or endorphins, which increase relaxation and the feeling of happiness. It has also been known to cause beneficial mechanical changes in the body.

Massage speeds up the overall healing process by helping to eliminate the buildup of toxins that occur after plastic surgery and increasing the circulation of blood to the affected area: bringing nutrients to both the skin and its underlying layers of tissue. Good circulation is a key in the recovery process and by encouraging a healthier blood flow massage can help to return nourishment and flexibility to the affected area. Massage therapy also helps build up the immune system, thus helping to speed up the overall healing. Clinical studies have indicated that massage can naturally increase the immune system's cytotoxic capacity—the activity level of the body's natural killer cells—and decrease the number of T-cells, which improves the body's immune functioning overall.

There are many different types of massage practiced today. For the purposes of recovery after cosmetic plastic surgery, I use three specific types of massage techniques to address issues you will experience at different stages of recovery. In this chapter, I first teach you how to perform lymphatic drainage massage, which is a gentle technique that facilitates a reduction in post-surgical swelling. In the upcoming chapters I instruct you on the second technique, a more aggressive form of massage that will help the tissue heal smoothly (getting rid of lumps) after procedures such as liposuction and breast augmentation. I then instruct you in the third technique, cross-friction massage, which addresses scar reduction.

While these tips and techniques are helpful and useful, please remember that massage should not be used until you receive approval from your surgeon.

What is the Lymphatic System?

The Lymphatic System

The lymphatic system is an intricate network of vessels and nodes functioning as a drainage and transport system. It aids the immune system in removing and destroying waste, debris, dead blood cells, pathogens, toxins, and cancer cells. The lymphatic system absorbs fats and fat-soluble vitamins from the digestive system and delivers these nutrients to the cells of the body. The lymphatic system also removes excess fluid, and waste products from cells.

The lymphatic system is known to be a transport system accompanying and closely associated with the blood's circulatory system. It plays a big role in our immune system.

The lymphatic system consists of two semi-independent parts: the lymphatic vessels and the lymphoid tissues and organs.

Lymphatic Vessels

The lymphatic vessels transport fluids that have escaped from the blood's vascular system back into the blood.

Lymphoid Tissues and Organs

The lymphoid organs house cells that play an essential role in the body's resistance to disease and overall immune defense. The lymphatic organs in the body are composed of lymph nodes, thymus glands, spleen, tonsils, and Peyer's patches.

For the purpose of teaching you lymphatic massage, there are only two areas of the lymphatic system that I will explain in detail: lymph nodes and lymphatic watersheds. These two things will affect how you perform the massage.

Lymph Nodes

Lymph nodes are bean-shaped nodules of tissue located along the vessels of the lymphatic system, notably in the neck, armpits, and groin. Lymph nodes filter foreign particles from lymph fluid. They help to protect against infection by killing bacteria and neutralizing toxins. Lymphocytes, one type of our immune system's white cells, use the lymph as a highway to all parts of the body.

Lymph is a clear, watery, yellowish fluid that originates in body tissues. It contains white blood cells and circulates throughout the lymphatic system, returning to the venous bloodstream through the thoracic duct. Lymph acts to remove bacteria and certain proteins from the tissues, transport fat from the small intestine, and supply mature lymphocytes to the blood.

There are approximately 600–700 lymph nodes in the human body. The majority of them are found in the abdomen, pelvis, and the head and neck region. The remainder are scattered about various parts of the body, including the armpit and chest areas. Each lymph node and lymph node group receives lymph from a specific region of the body.

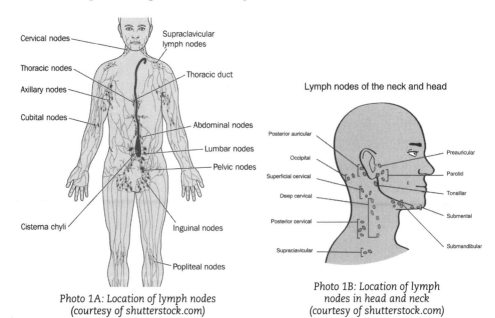

Photo 1A: Location of lymph nodes
(courtesy of shutterstock.com)

Photo 1B: Location of lymph nodes in head and neck
(courtesy of shutterstock.com)

Why are lymph nodes important in massage?

These regions are important to know for your lymphatic massage because when massaging a body part to get rid of swelling, you first massage the area's lymph node(s). This will wake up the lymph nodes—the place where swelling is filtered out of your body. For example, if you are massaging out swelling in the thigh, you start by massaging the lymph nodes in the groin.

Lymphatic Watersheds

The skin is broken up into regions called lymphatic watersheds. Just like a continental divide, the boundaries between these regions represent the direction of lymphatic flow in a particular body area. For the purposes of lymphatic massage, these boundaries deter-

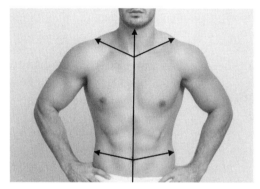

Photo 2: The lines mark the boundaries of the lymphatic watersheds

mine which direction you will massage. It is extremely important to determine the correct direction for your massage strokes during lymphatic massage.

Direction of Flow

Whatever areas you are massaging, the lymph, or swelling, must be sent towards the group of lymph nodes responsible for drainage of that area. The direction of flow is determined by the watershed boundaries.

In the images to the right, follow the arrows to see in which direction you should massage.

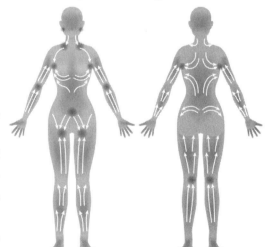

Photo 3: The direction of flow is the direction in which you should massage (courtesy of shutterstock.com)

Rules for the Torso

Rule 1: The vertical line going down the middle of the trunk separates the body into two halves. You always massage starting from the middle and going outwards.

Rule 2: The horizontal line at the belly button separates the torso into two parts: top and bottom. Everything above this line gets massaged toward the armpits. Everything below this line gets massaged toward the groin.

Rule 3: The horizontal line at the collarbone separates the chest and neck area into two parts. Everything above that line gets massaged down toward the line. Everything below that line gets massaged towards the armpits.

Rules for the Legs

Rule 1: Always massage the legs toward the groin, never towards the feet.

Rule 2: Always massage from the inner thigh towards the outer thigh.

Rule 3: Always massage the thigh the from the knee towards the groin.

Rule 4: Massage the lower leg from the ankle towards the knee.

Rule 5: Massage the foot from the toes toward the ankle.

Rules for the Arms

Rule 1: Always massage the arm toward the armpit, never towards the hand.

Rule 2: Always massage from hand towards the wrist toward the elbow towards the shoulder.

Rules for the Face

Rule 1: Imagine a line going down (vertical) the center of the face. Always massage out towards the ear, away from the line.

Rule 2: Always massage down the neck towards the collarbone.

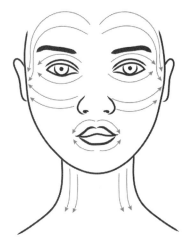

**Lymphatic drainage
face massage**

*Photo 4: Lymphatic watersheds of the face
(courtesy of shutterstock.com)*

What is Lymphatic Drainage Massage?

Lymphatic drainage massage is a gentle technique that stimulates the movement and absorption of lymph. It is commonly used for lymphedema patients, post-surgical patients, and most injuries that result in swelling. It is not a typical massage of the skin and muscles, but rather a stretching of the skin to increase movement of fluid to the swollen area.

Manual lymph drainage (MLD), now commonly called lymphatic drainage massage, was invented in 1932 by Emil Vodder, Ph.D., M.T. in Cannes, France. As a massage therapist, his clients generally sought out his services to soothe their muscle aches and pains during chronic colds. Vodder noticed that direct, intuitive, and gentle manipulation on swollen lymph nodes caused rapid improvement in muscle pain during colds. These findings inspired him to develop therapy based on ancient drawings of lymphatic anatomy. The technique is employed using gentle, subtle hand movements.

Purpose

As mentioned before, lymphatic drainage massage is a therapy involving the lymphatic system. The lymphatic system is responsible for absorbing and carrying waste products away from connective tissues back to the bloodstream. The waste includes dead cells, fatty acids, proteins, and also viruses and bacteria. During the transportation process, the lymphatic system is cleaned, filtered, and concentrated with many immune reactions occurring in the lymph nodes. When there is disruption to lymph nodes because of surgery, the lymphatic system cannot carry waste and fluid away from the injured area. As a result, swelling happens.

After swelling has set in, massage is an effective technique used to reduce swelling and open channels to allow excess fluids and waste to drain from the affected area. Lymphatic massage is a specialized type of gentle massage that is designed to aid in lymphatic circulation to help your body's lymphatic system work properly again.

What Is the Role of Lymphatic Drainage Massage After Plastic Surgery?

Lymphatic drainage massage improves lymph flow and accelerates the removal of the waste products accumulated during surgery, and thus speeds up the healing process. Lymphatic massage mimics the pulse and flow within the lymph system: It decongests the tissue and therefore allows blood to flow freely, thus reducing swelling and stimulating the immune system.

Lymphatic massage can be used after many different types of plastic surgery, but it is now most commonly used after liposuction procedures. Nearly all liposuction procedures produce some degree of swelling in the areas on which the surgery is performed.

What exactly is the cause of swelling in liposuction patients? In some instances, swelling is the result of the trauma that is inflicted on the remaining fat cells by cutting movements that were made too aggressively by the surgeon during the procedure. Swelling is more likely to occur when liposuction is performed on the lower portion of the body. Individuals who have had previous liposuction surgeries are also more likely to develop swelling because repeated procedures, particularly on the same area, are more prone to additional swelling due to the buildup of scar tissue. Lymphatic massage helps to alleviate soreness and reduce swelling in these target areas.

When a patient performs lymphatic massage on himself or herself, it is called simple lymphatic drainage (SLD). In the rest of this chapter I teach you how to do SLD.

When Can Lymphatic Drainage Massage Begin?

Clearance to begin lymphatic massage should be determined by your doctor based on your individual status, but usually it begins when the doctor allows you to begin to take off your compression garment or bandages for a brief period of time. The benefit of lymphatic massage early in your recovery is to reduce swelling and inflammation and prevent tissue fibrosis from developing.

How Often Should Lymphatic Drainage Massage Be Performed?

Ideally, lymphatic massage should be performed at least once daily for at least 15–20 minutes, directly preceding your regular exercise program, and should be followed by skin care and compression therapy, i.e. correctly wearing your garment.

Contraindications for Lymphatic Drainage Massage

Please consult your plastic surgeon and get clearance before beginning lymphatic drainage massage. If you have any of the general contraindications listed below, you should not have lymphatic massage.

General Contraindications

If swelling is solely due to cardiac failure or the patient is not taking the appropriate medication to treat the heart failure

Severe kidney disease as lymphatic drainage massage will put stress on the kidneys

Acute infection of any type, anywhere in your body

Acute episode of deep vein thrombosis (DVT).

Once the DVT has been medically managed and is stable and the patient has been medically cleared by their doctor, massage may begin.

Contraindications for Massage of the Neck

Observe all general contraindications

Cardiac arrhythmia

Hypersensitive carotid sinus, which could affect blood pressure and heart rhythm

Hyperthyroidism, as massage could release the excess thyroid hormones into the bloodstream.

Patients over 60 should be cautious as massage could loosen and release built-up cholesterol plaques located in the arteries.

Contraindications for Massage of the Face

Observe all general contraindications

Any inflammatory process of the face, to avoid spreading infection

Contraindications for Massage of the Deep Abdomen

Observe general contraindications

Pregnancy

Abdominal aortic aneurysm

Diverticulitis or diverticulosis

Severe arteriosclerosis

Inflammatory bowel disease, i.e. Crohn's disease or ulcerative colitis

Irradiation of the abdominal region

Pelvic deep vein thrombosis

Presence of clot-prevention devices, i.e. IVC filter

Unexplained pain

Menstruation (more of a precaution than contraindication)

Tips for Lymphatic Drainage Massage

Drink plenty of water before and after your treatment to increase your results. Water is an internal hydrant. It keeps the skin moist from the inside out.

If your skin is dry, use a small amount of lotion before massage. Allow the lotion to absorb into the skin before you start. A lot of lotion should not be used for this technique—slippery skin may be good for a Swedish massage but it's not good here!

Self-massage should always be pain-free. If you're experiencing pain, you may be doing something wrong—reread the steps, and try again!

Self-massage may be done while seated or lying down. Never strain your shoulders, neck, arm, or hand when doing self-massage.

Technique for Lymphatic Drainage Massage

Use your hands, not your fingertips! Hands allow more contact with the skin, and they should be flat, soft, and relaxed. I always tell my patients to imagine their hands are like a spatula and you are icing a cake. You want your hands to move smoothly and evenly across the body, not gripping separated fingers, which would cause "tracks in the icing of your cake."

Try to find the most comfortable position for your hands without straining your wrists too much.

Pressure should be just enough to stretch the skin. You do not want to slide or rub the skin. Gently stretch the skin as far as it goes naturally, and then release.

The rhythm of your massage strokes should be slow. The rate of strokes should be done in a one-second rhythm: massage (count, one Mississippi), then stop, then massage (count, one Mississippi), then stop.

What You Need to Know Before You Start

Lymph nodes are always massaged before body parts in order to wake them up. Lymph nodes are the key to filtering the swelling out of your body.

Always begin with a pre-treatment massage—this means you should treat the central part of the body before you treat the limbs. This causes a suction effect like a vacuum cleaner sucks up dust and debris, bringing lymph fluid to the center of the body so it can be flushed out.

The direction and order of the massage are very important. First, the areas of the body where nodes are concentrated (neck, arm pit, or groin) are stimulated in order to ready them to receive more fluid. Then the strokes begin close to the nodes, moving fluid toward them with slow and rhythmic strokes.

When massaging your limbs, never massage away from the body. This means never massage towards your hands when massaging your arms—massage towards your armpit. This also means never massage towards your feet when massaging your legs—massage towards your groin.

It is common to have to urinate after lymphatic massage treatment because fluid is leaving your body.

Nausea and dizziness are sometimes a common side effect after lymphatic massage. If you experience nausea or dizziness after the massage treatment, this means you successfully expelled a large amount of fluid during your treatment—this is great! These symptoms are temporary and should resolve shortly after they occur. Rest, drink some orange juice and allow your body to re-adjust until symptoms resolve.

When performing lymphatic massage, it is important to remember that the pressure of your hands on your skin should be very light. If you can feel your muscles underneath your fingers, then you are pressing too hard and going too deep.

Lymphatic Massage Sequences

Pre-treatment Massage

The following four steps will be performed at the start of every treatment session, no matter what area of the body you are working on.

Step 1. Deep breathing

Deep breathing is done by contracting the diaphragm.

Begin by placing both hands flat on your belly, over your diaphragm.

Inhale slowly—breathe deeply through your nose, allowing your stomach to expand into your hands.

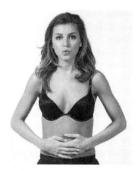

Photo 5: Deep breathing

As air enters your lungs, your abdomen—not your chest wall—should expand outwards.

Breathe out slowly through pursed lips, allowing your stomach to flatten.

Repeat five times with a short rest between each breath to avoid dizziness.

Step 2. Collarbone (clavicle)

Place the bottom of your second (index) and third (middle) fingers on either side of your neck just above your collarbone.

Stroke down towards your collarbone and inward toward your neck. Stretch the skin just as far as it naturally goes. This stroke would look like two "J" strokes facing one another.

This technique can be applied on both sides at the same time or on one side at a time.

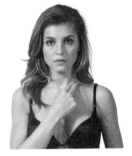

If doing both sides at the same time, you may find it more comfortable to cross your arms while you do this stroke.

Repeat 15 times.

Photo 6: Collarbone massage

Step 3. Side of neck

Place the bottom of your hands on either side of your neck just under your ears and gently stretch the skin down towards your collarbone and release.

Keep a slow and rhythmic pace.

Repeat this stroke 10 to 15 times.

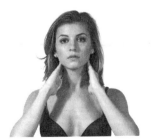
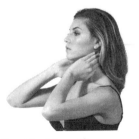

Photo 7A-B: Massaging the side of the neck

Step 4. Back of neck

Place the bottom of your hands on the back of your neck just below your hairline on either side of your spine.

Stretch the skin towards the spine and then down toward base of neck and release.

Repeat 10 to 15 times.

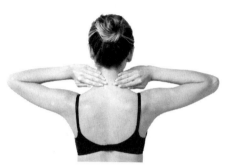

Photo 8: Massaging the back of the neck

Abdominal Massage Treatment

The following steps massage the lymphatic vessels of the deep abdomen, located beneath the abdominal muscles. These treatments are used after liposuction of the abdomen, abdominoplasty, body lift, breast implants, or any abdominal surgery.

Step 1. Pre-treatment massage

Perform in this order: collarbone, side of neck, back of neck, and deep breathing, all as described above.

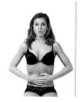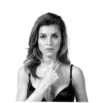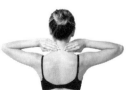

Photo 9A-D: Steps for abdominal pre-treatment massage

Step 2. Clockwise circles

Place your hand on the center of your abdomen, between your rib cage and navel.

With deep pressure, gently push inward and upward, the up and down rhythm is like the motions of a wave.

Next, move your hand to positions the starred positions, performing five repetitions at each position).

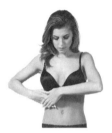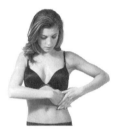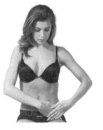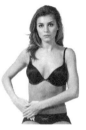

Photo 10A-D: Position for clockwise circles

Step 3. Abdominal "V"

Place your hands flat on both sides of your lower abdomen, forming the letter "V."

Push inward and then upward on a diagonal, towards the belly button in a wave.

The movement is a three-second deep stretch.

Release for three seconds and then repeat four times.

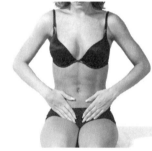

Photo 11: Hand position for abdominal "V"

Chest Massage Treatment

Chest massage is used following breast implants, pectoral implants, liposuction of the abdomen/flanks, body lift, or any upper body surgery. This technique can also be used before massage treatment of the arms for additional benefits.

Step 1. Pre-treatment massage

Perform in this order: collarbone, side of neck, back of neck, and deep breathing, all as described above.

 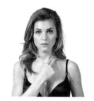 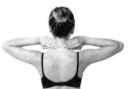

Photo 12A-D: Order of steps for chest pre-treatment massage

Step 2. Armpit lymph nodes

To prepare to redirect fluid from the chest area, you gently pump your hand in the center of your underarm by placing your palm against your armpit.

Knead your palm firmly in a counterclockwise circle.

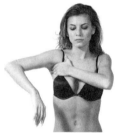

Pressure is applied with the flat surfaces of your fingers and palm, and is directed downward, deep into the armpit.

Perform this in each armpit about 10 to 15 times.

Photo 13: Stimulating the axillary nodes

Step 3. Chest

Place your fingers on your breast bone (sternum), in the middle of your chest above one breast.

Push your hand gently towards your opposite armpit, stretching your skin, as far as it naturally goes, and then release.

Repeat this motion 10 to 15 times, slowly moving your hand placement closer towards the armpit.

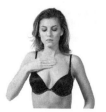 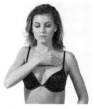 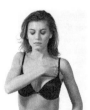

Photo 14A-C: Chest massage

Arm Massage Treatment

This is used after arm lift, liposuction of the arm, neck lift, and any surgery which results in residual swelling of the upper extremities.

Step 1. Pre-treatment massage

Perform in this order: collarbone, side of neck, back of neck, and deep breathing, all as described above.

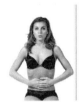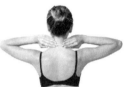

Photo 15A-D: Order of steps for pretreatment massage of arm

Step 2. Armpit lymph nodes

If the left arm is swollen, massage the left armpit (underarm).

If the right arm is swollen, massage the right armpit (underarm).

If both are swollen, massage under both.

Perform in a circular motion.

The pressure is applied with the flats of fingers and palm and is directed downward, deep into the armpit.

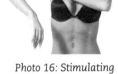

Photo 16: Stimulating the axillary nodes

Step 3. Upper arm

Lymphatic fluid in the upper arm normally flows into the underarm. You want to direct the fluid to the axillary lymph nodes.

Starting with your shoulder, gently massage towards your neck. If it is not too much of a strain on your wrist, stroke across the back of your shoulder to your neck.

Try to gently stretch your skin towards your neck, then release. Repeat 15 times.

Massage your whole upper arm from the inside of your arm to the top of your upper arm.

Repeat 15 times.

Now massage from the back of your arm to the top of your upper arm, stretching your skin, and then release.

Repeat 15 times.

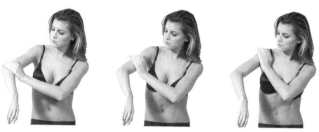

Photo 17A-C: Steps in upper arm massage— shoulder to neck, inside of arm to top of arm, and back of arm to top of arm

Step 4. Forearm and the hand

Gently massage your forearm from the wrist to the elbow.

Next start with your fingers and go over the top of the hand.

Finish by going back up the entire arm over wrist, forearm, elbow, upper arm, and then shoulder.

Gently stretching your skin, push fluid upwards and then release.

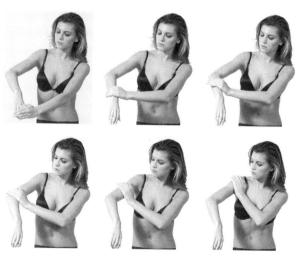

Photo 18A-F: Massaging hand all the way up to the shoulder

Leg Massage Treatment

This treatment is used after liposuction of the thigh, knee, or lower leg; calf augmentation; thigh lift; or any surgery performed on the leg.

Step 1. Pre-treatment massage

Perform in this order: collarbone, side of neck, back of neck, and deep breathing, all as described above.

 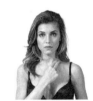 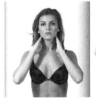 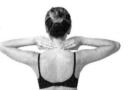

Photo 19A-D: Order of steps for pre-treatment massage of the leg

Step 2. Groin lymph nodes and outer thigh lymph nodes

Lie on your back. Bend your leg slightly and then place your hand on the angle that forms between your leg and pelvis. Place your fingertips on this crease. Your hand is placed just below the hipbone, but closer to your private area.

Make circles for two to three minutes, directing the pressure toward your belly.

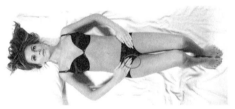

Photo 20A: Massaging the groin lymph nodes

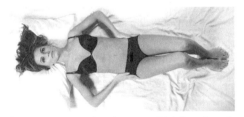

Photo 20B: Massaging the outer thigh lymph nodes

Step 3. Outside of upper thigh

Make stationary circles with the back of your hand and fingers in several places on the outside of your thigh and hip.

Pressure is directed toward your waist.

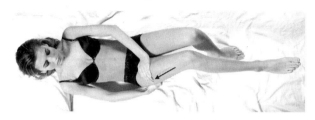

Photo 21: Massaging the outside of the upper thigh

Step 4. Inside of upper thigh

Starting on the inside of your upper thigh, make stationary circles and massage towards the outside of your thigh.

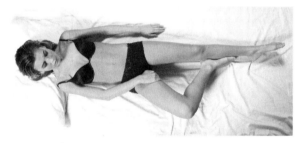

Photo 22: Massaging inside of upper thigh

Step 5. Thigh just above knee

Make stationary circles just above your knee, starting on the inside and moving towards the outside of your thigh.

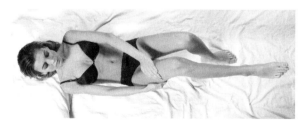

Photo 23: Massaging the thigh above the knee

Step 6. Lower outer thigh

Make stationary circles with your hand flat against the outside of your thigh.

Start just above the knee and stroke upward towards the hip.

Pressure is directed from the knee towards the hip

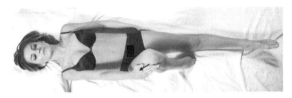

Photo 24: Massaging the lower outer thigh

Step 7. Repeat outside of upper thigh

Make stationary circles with the back of your hand and fingers in several places on the outside of your thigh and hip.

Pressure is directed toward your waist.

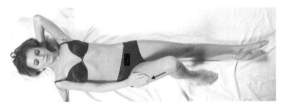

Photo 25: Massaging the outside of the upper thigh

Step 8. Back of knee

Make stationary circles with the flats of your hands, behind your knee.

Pressure is directed gently upwards toward the thigh.

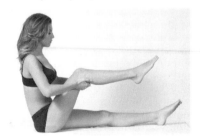

Photo 26: Massaging the back of your knee

Step 9. Outside and inside of knee

Make stationary circles with the flats of your fingers, gently stroking the inside and outside of your knee.

Pressure is directed towards the thigh.

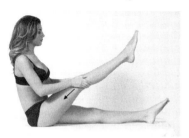

Photo 27: Massaging the inside
and outside of the knee

Step 10. Lower leg

Make stationary circles with the flat of your hand on the inner and outer surface of your lower leg (your calf).

Direct the strokes upwards towards your knee.

Massage the entire area from your ankle to your knee.

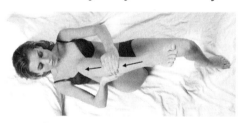

Photo 28: Massaging your lower leg

Step 11. Top of foot

Make stationary circles on the top of your foot, stroking towards your ankle.

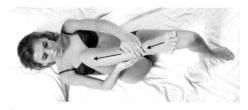

Photo 29: Massage on top of foot and move upwards

Step 12. Entire leg

Repeat strokes, going from foot, ankle back up your entire leg to your groin.

Face Massage Treatment

This is used after rhinoplasty, facelift, chin augmentation, lip augmentation, and forehead or brow lift.

Use the photo below (30) to guide you when performing the massage techniques.

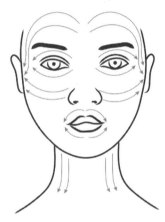

**Lymphatic drainage
face massage**

*Photo 30: Watershed regions of the face and neck,
with arrows showing correct direction for massage strokes
(courtesy of shutterstock.com)*

Step 1. Pre-treatment massage

Perform in this order: collarbone, side of neck, back of neck, and deep breathing, all as described above.

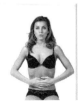   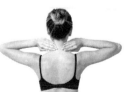

Photo 31A-D: Order of steps for face pre-treatment massage

Step 2. Under jaw

Place your flat on the soft tissue under your jaw close to your ear.

Stroke under your jaw down towards your collarbone.

Repeat strokes covering the entire neck area from the jaw downwards.

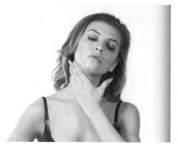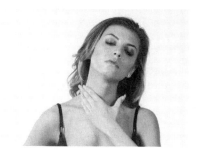

Photo 32A-B: Massage under jaw down towards collarbone

Step 3. Chin

Place the pads of your fingers on your chin, below your lower lip. Gently make circles, pulling your skin in the direction of your ear five times.

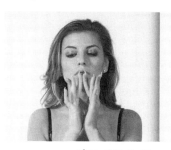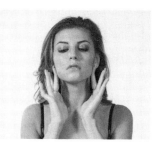

Photo 33A-B: Massage from the chin,
along the lower face, towards the ear.

Step 4. Upper lip

Place the pads of your fingers below your upper lip. Gently make circles that pull your skin outwards in the direction of your ear five times.

Repeat this in two different places, just to the side of your mouth and just above your upper lip.

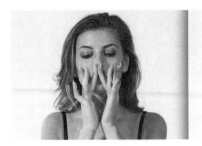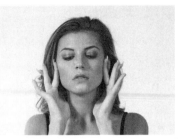

Photo 34A-B: Massage from the upper lip,
along the mid-face, towards the ear.

Step 5. Nose

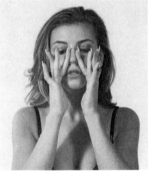

Place the pads of your fingers just
to the side of your nostrils. Gently
make circles that pull your skin in the
direction of your ear five times.

Repeat this in two different places,
just to the side of the bridge of your
nose and right below the inside edge
of your eye.

Photo 35: Massage from
the bridge of the nose
towards the outside
of the nose.

Step 6. Cheeks

Start at the sides of your nose, just under your eyes, and
massage out towards your ears.

Repeat this in order to massage the entire cheek.

Repeat this just below the cheekbones as well.

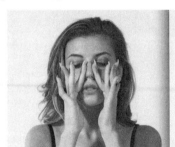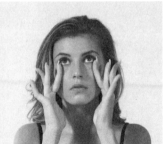

Photo 36A-B: Massage from the sides of the nose,
along the mid-face, towards the ear.

Step 7. Eyelids

Place all your fingertips just below your eye and stretch your skin gently toward your ears five times. Repeat above the eyelids.

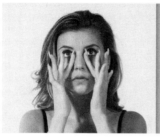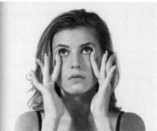

Photo 37A-B: Massage from the corner of your eye, under your eyelids, towards the ear.

Step 8. Eyebrows

Place all your fingertips just below your eye and stretch your skin gently toward your ears five times. Repeat this in two different places along your eyebrows, moving from nose toward your ears.

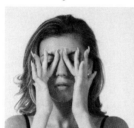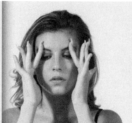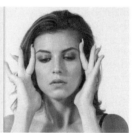

Photo 38A-C: Massage from bridge of your nose, across the eyebrows, towards the ear.

Step 9. Lower Forehead

Place the fingers of both hands on the center of your forehead and gently stretch down and outwards towards your ears five times.

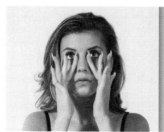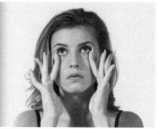

Photo 39A-B: Massage from the center of your lower forehead outward, towards your ear.

Step 10. Upper forehead

Gently place your hands at the top of your forehead at the hairline.

Putting pressure with the flats of your hands, gently pull from the center out towards your ears five times.

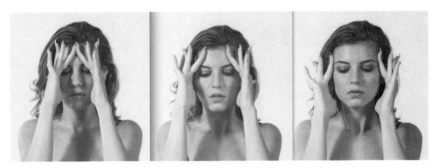

Photo 40A-C: Massage from the center of your upper forehead outward, towards your ear.

Chapter 11

How to Reduce Lumps

Adhesions are bands of scar tissue that form due to tissue trauma and as part of the healing process. This tissue trauma occurs after certain plastic surgery procedures, most commonly after liposuction and breast augmentation. The damaged tissue is weakened and vulnerable until fully healed. So, to prevent re-injury the body responds by protecting the area with extra tissue—scar tissue. It is called an adhesion because the scar tissue binds, or adheres, to the surrounding tissue. The problem is that after the damaged site has healed, the scar tissue remains there. Adhesions can restrict motion, cause pain, and result in a lumpy appearance. A combination of massage and exercise can reduce these adhesions.

Massage after Breast Augmentation

The purpose of massage after breast augmentation is to prevent the formation of lumps in the form of excessive scar tissue, both in the incision and around the implant. It is important to maintain the soft feeling of your breasts and not develop a stereotypical rock hard "boob job." Your body's natural response to the presence of a foreign body—the implant—is to stimulate the growth of scar tissue. Since your body experiences the incision as an injury, it sends fiber cells to the area of the incision to repair the damage.

Massage after breast augmentation surgery can help speed up the healing of the incision, reduce the risk of capsular contracture, and help produce soft, natural-looking breasts. Massage of the implants is recommended by some surgeons, but not all. Those who do recommend it feel that it reduces the growth of a scar tissue capsule around the implant. Keeping scar tissue at a minimum helps keep the breasts soft and flexible, and prevents the implant from moving to an undesired position.

Whether massage is a good idea after breast augmentation surgery depends on the type of implant used and your physician's preference. Massage is not recommended for textured implants.

Capsular Contracture After Breast Augmentation Surgery

What is Capsular Contracture?

Capsular contracture refers to a hardening of the breast pocket and scar tissue around breast implant. When this happens, the breast implant is compressed, causing the breast to feel too hard and become misshapen. Symptoms of capsular contracture include hardness, swelling, and pain in your breast. Capsular contracture can be very painful and should be addressed as soon as possible.

Capsular contracture affects approximately five percent of women who have breast augmentation, but the specific rate of contracture is unknown.

Capsular contracture is the most frequent condition that leads to re-operation after breast implant surgery. A capsular contracture typically develops three months after surgery, though it can develop at any time. Factors associated with capsular contracture formation include infection, hematoma, silicone bleed, and individual predisposition to hypertrophic scarring (big thick scar).

Grading capsular contracture

For over 30 years, the Baker system has been a widespread, four-tier scale for grading capsule thickening or contracture.

Grade I. The breast has normal softness and appears natural in size and shape.

Grade II. The breast is a little firm but appears normal.

Grade III. The breast is firm and appears abnormal.

Grade IV. The breast is hard, painful to the touch, and appears abnormal.

Preventing capsular contracture

Prevention of capsular contraction is a joint effort between you and your surgeon. The technique your surgeon utilizes, the type of implant chosen, and placement of the implant are all factors that may affect the chances of developing a capsular contracture. Factors that you, as the patient, have greater control over include wearing your postoperative compression garment, following the specified exercise program, and performing post-operative massage.

Massage to Prevent Capsular Contracture

Regular breast massage in the first six months following surgery can reduce the risk for capsular contracture by moving your implants so that they can move freely within the implant pocket and retain the contour and symmetry of your breasts.

I teach my patients that implant massage helps to create a pocket that is larger than the implant itself. This helps the implant move around naturally inside its pocket and will create natural shape and motion, like a normal breast.

Breast massage also functions to some extent as a breast self-exam. Two studies found that women who developed potentially cancerous breast lumps found them earlier if they regularly massaged and felt their implants—proving that breast massage can be potentially life-saving.

When to Perform Breast Massage

Doctors typically recommend that you wait until after your one-week post-op visit to begin massage—get approval from your doctor before beginning any massage protocol.

Perform the following techniques, as shown below, while lying down, at least twice each day for the first three months following surgery. While this may be uncomfortable when you first begin to perform the exercises, it is very important that you stick to them. After three months, if your breasts feel soft and the implants are moving freely, you may reduce your exercise and only perform your exercises one time a day.

After every day during the first year, you may perform your exercises once per day or every other day.

When Not to Perform Breast Massage

When your doctor advises against it

If you begin to experience any sharp pain in your breast

Hot or flushed skin over your breast

Severe spontaneous tightening or hardness within your breast implants

Severe pain to touch

Pus coming out from the incision or the nipple

Bloody drainage

Incision around the breast is separated and opening

Immediately stop the exercises and contact your doctor as soon as possible.

Massage Techniques

Technique 1

With your bra off, cup your breast directly under your nipple. The palm should push inward—not up—and then roll up tightly against the chest wall. This causes the implant to rise upwards—watch for the implant to slide up as in the right photograph.

To make sure the breasts are at the same level as when they were initially positioned, look in the mirror as you push both breasts.

Repeat this on each breast 10 times, holding for 10 seconds, three times a day.

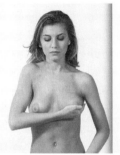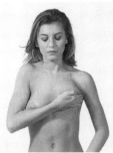

Photo 1A-B: Massage technique 1 after augmentation—cupping (left) and rolling (right)

Technique 2

This downward massage can be done less frequently as the implant settles over the weeks after surgery.

To make sure the breasts are at the same level as when they were initially positioned, look in the mirror as you push both breasts.

Repeat this on each breast 10 times, holding for 10 seconds, three times a day.

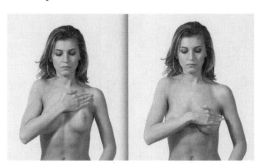

Photo 2A-B: Massage technique 2 after augmentation—downward push

Technique 3

This technique is used to address the sides of the implant.

Cup the outsides of your breast with your palms and simultaneously bring them together.

To make sure the breasts are evenly coming together, look in the mirror as you push both breasts.

Repeat this on each breast 10 times, holding for 10 seconds, three times a day.

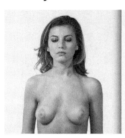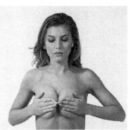

Photo 3A-B: Massage technique 3 after augmentation—resting breast position and side cupping/pushing breasts together

Technique 4

Massage over the entire breast in a circular pattern starting at the top.

Make a large circle clockwise.

Start the second circle at the top, but just below your original starting point.

Each time you complete a circle and start again, you should be getting closer to the nipple. Your last circle should be around the nipple.

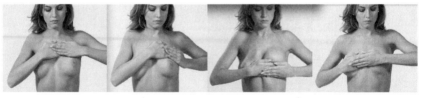

Photo 4A-D: Massage technique 4 after augmentation—massage in a circular motion around the entire breast.

Massage after Fat Removal Surgery

Have you ever seen a picture of a celebrity who had liposuction? I'm sure that if you have, the picture you saw was of a lumpy and rippled stomach. This may not be because of poor surgical skills, but instead due to scar tissue formation during the healing process. This could have most likely been prevented with proper postoperative care and massage.

Surgical liposuction is a form of surgery sucking out the excess fat from the layer below the skin—a tube is inserted under the skin and fat is drawn out.

First Phase of Massage after Liposuction

The first phase of massage after liposuction is lymphatic drainage massage, as described in Chapter 10. In this chapter I am going to focus on the second phase of massage after liposuction.

Second Phase of Massage after Liposuction

This massage gets into the deeper layers of muscle tissues and break down any muscle adhesion that can be felt. The focus of the second phase of massage after liposuction includes:

- Reducing skin rippling and adhesions
- Softening tissue
- Relieving pain
- Increasing range of motion
- Renewing skin elasticity
- Smoothing out lumps and bumps

Getting a professional massage from someone who can help you break down the adhesions is beneficial. If you are unable to get a professional massage, here are self-massage techniques to perform daily:

Abdomen

Using the pads of your fingers, start by pressing *firmly* right above your belly button. Make a small circle around the belly button, and then gradually make the circle bigger as you continue.

Apply *firm, deep pressure* all around the abdomen. Follow the outline that you traced with your strokes in step one. Use one hand on top of the other, or the palm of just one hand, and apply deep pressure. When you hit a lumpy spot, focus the strokes over that area. Press firmly downward and work over that area with small circles.

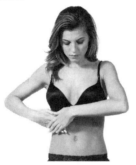 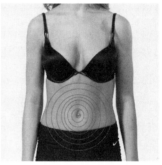

Photo 5A-B: *Pattern for massage after abdominal liposuction*

Arms

Circle technique

Place your forearm on a supported surface—consider using a table with a rolled towel under your arm, so your elbow is free.

Starting underneath your arm slightly above the elbow, apply deep pressure with the pads of your four fingers. Allow your thumb to rest comfortably on the top part of your arm.

Gradually perform small circles in a straight path towards your armpit.

Move your hand, repeating this pattern, until you have massage the entire surface of the upper arm.

When you hit a lumpy spot, focus the strokes over that area. Press firmly downward and work over that area with small circles. Make sure to not just get the top of the arm, get all areas, including underneath.

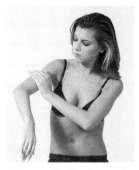

Photo 6: Deep Massage in circular motions up the arm

Pinch technique

Another technique to address the lumpy areas is to pinch the area gently between your thumb and your pointer/index and middle fingers, and then knead the spot.

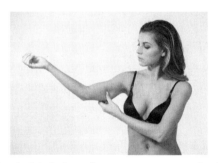

Photo 7: The pinch technique of upper arm massage after liposuction

Back

It's tough to reach your own back for a massage, but try using a ball to do the job.

Place the ball between your back and the wall.

Carefully apply your body weight against the wall, until you get the desired pressure.

Rock your body to move the ball around your back.

A smaller ball will provide a more concentrated amount of pressure and a bigger ball will provide more diffuse pressure.

Try both sizes of balls to achieve both results.

Another household item can help you with the sides of your back. Grab your grandma's rolling pin and use it on your flanks and sides. If you prefer you can purchase a massage roller as seen in the photo. Start near the hip and roll up towards your ribcage. Repeat this motion, moving the roller further back each time.

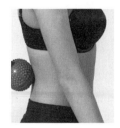

Photo 8: Using a ball to help perform back massage after liposuction

Thighs

Start by lying on your back with your hip and knee flexed (see below).

Using both hands, cup behind your knee and apply firm pressure.

Begin kneading your thigh in the direction towards your buttocks.

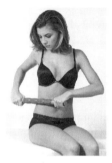

Photo 9: Using a roller to massage back after liposuction

Repeat this massage on the sides, back, and top of your thigh.

Grab and lift large sections of your thigh with both hands.

Again, work your way from the knee to the top of the leg.

Take a rolling pin from your kitchen and use it to smooth out your thigh. The rolling pin is placed behind the knee and rolled towards the groin. Repeat over all areas of the thigh. Rolling over bony prominences, i.e. your hip bone, may cause discomfort.

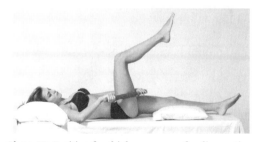

Photo 10: Position for thigh massage after liposuction, this view showing use of a roller

Exercises to Reduce Lumps

The following exercises are for the second phase of recovery, after your incisions have healed. Typically, these exercises can begin three to four weeks after surgery. Always ask your doctor when it is safe to begin this exercise program. Always stop any exercise if you are experiencing pain.

Exercises after Abdominal Surgery

The following seven exercises are to be performed during the second phase of recovery after any procedure on the abdomen, i.e. abdominoplasty, body lift, or liposuction. The purpose of these exercises is to break down adhesions and increase range of motion. Typically start these exercises 3-4 weeks post surgery date.

Lumbar rotation lying down

Lie on one side with one hip and knee bent.

Position your lower arm straight in front of you.

Position your other hand behind your neck.

Twist your trunk and shoulders backward.

Return to the start position.

Perform two sets of 10 repetitions twice a day.

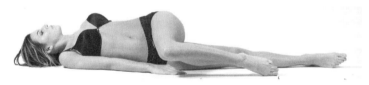

Photo 11: Lumbar rotation lying down

Standing side bend

Stand upright with good posture: feet shoulder width apart and arms at your side.

Slowly bend to one side, reaching toward the ground.

Return upright and repeat to the other side.

Perform two sets of 10 repetitions twice a day.

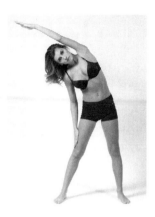

Photo 12: Standing side bend

Standing rotation

Stand upright, shoulders back, with good posture.

Place your hands on your hips.

Slowly rotate to one side, not moving your hands, leading with your elbow.

Return to center and repeat to the other side.

Perform two sets of 10 repetitions twice a day.

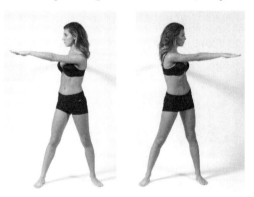

Photo 13A-B: Standing trunk rotation in standing

Prone press-ups

Begin lying on your stomach, with your hands flat, under your shoulders.

Slowly press up, extending your elbows straight.

Make sure your hips are pressed firmly to the ground.
For added stretch, look up towards the ceiling.
Hold for eight seconds.
Perform two sets of 10 repetitions, twice a day.

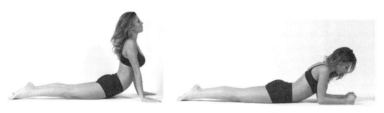

Photo 14A-B: Prone press up in standing

Standing extension

Stand upright, shoulders back, with good posture.
Place your hands on the back of your hips.
Slowly extend backwards, not moving your hands.
Hold at end range for five seconds.
For an added stretch, look up toward the ceiling.
Return to the start position then repeat.
Perform two sets of 10 repetitions twice a day.

Photo 15A-B: Standing back extension

Exercises after Arm Surgery

The following exercises are to be performed during the second phase of recovery after any procedure on the arms, i.e. arm lift or liposuction. The purpose of these exercises is to break down adhesions and increase range of motion. Typically start these exercises 3-4 weeks post surgery date.

Triceps dips

Start facing away from a chair, bench, or step. Make sure the object does not move.

Place your hand on the surface, keeping your legs either straight or bent.

Bend your elbows and then straighten.

Perform two sets of 10 repetitions twice a day.

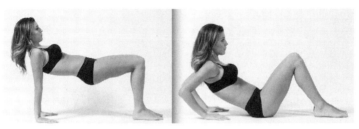

Photo 16A-B: Triceps dips

Push-ups

Get into a plank position with hands planted directly under the shoulders, slightly wider than shoulder width apart, and elbows extended.

Ground your toes into the floor or rest on your knees.

Lower to the ground by bending your elbows, then extend and push up.

Perform two sets of 10 repetitions twice a day.

Triceps stretch

Raise one arm straight overhead next to your ear, and then bend your forearm.

Grasp elbow overhead with other hand.

Pull elbow back and toward head.

Hold stretch for eight seconds.

Repeat with opposite arm.

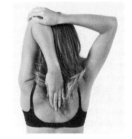

Photo 17: Triceps stretch

Perform two sets of 10 repetitions twice a day.

Cross body arm stretch

Stand grasping your elbow with your other hand as shown.

Pull the elbow and arm across your chest so that you feel a stretch.

Hold for eight seconds.

Repeat with opposite arm.

Perform two sets of 10 repetitions twice a day.

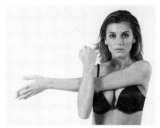

Photo 18: Cross body
arm stretch

Exercises after Back and Flank Surgery

The following exercises are to be performed during the second phase of recovery after any procedure on the back or flank area, i.e. body lift or liposuction. The purpose of these exercises is to break down adhesions and increase range of motion. Typically start these exercises 3-4 weeks post surgery date.

Child's pose

Begin by kneeling on the floor.

Bend forward with trunk, bending head and chin to your chest.

Reach forward placing your hands on the floor.

Sit back on your heels.

Hold for five seconds. Return to start position and repeat.

Perform two sets of 10 repetitions twice a day.

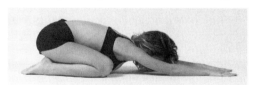

Photo 19: Child's pose

Child's pose with side bend

Assume child's pose.

Then bring your arms to one side, creating a bend at your waist.

Hold for five seconds. Return to start position and repeat to opposite side.

Perform two sets of 10 repetitions twice a day.

Forward bend

Stand upright with good posture: feet together or shoulder width apart.

Slowly roll down, bending at the hips, reaching toward the ground.

Hold for eight seconds then return upright.

Perform two sets of 10 repetitions twice a day.

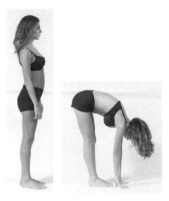

Photo 20A-B: Forward bend

Sitting forward bend at 45 degrees

Sit upright with good posture, feet together.
Rotate your body 45 degrees.
Then slowly roll down, bend at the hips, reaching toward the ground.
Hold for eight seconds then return upright.
Repeat on the other side.
Perform two sets of 10 repetitions twice a day.

Exercises after Buttock Surgery

The following exercises are to be performed during the second phase of recovery after any procedure on the buttocks, i.e. buttock augmentation or liposuction. The purpose of these exercises is to break down adhesions and increase range of motion. Typically start these exercises 3-4 weeks post surgery date.

Bridging

Lie on back with knees bent.
Lift buttocks off the floor.
Return to start position.
Perform two sets of 10 repetitions twice a day.

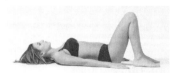 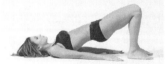

Photos 21A-B: Bridging

Bridging with ball

Lie on back with knees bent and feet on top of a large ball.

Lift buttocks off the floor and bring ball towards you.

Lower your hips as you return the ball to the start position.

Perform two sets of 10 repetitions twice a day.

Buttock press

Begin lying on your stomach.

With your knee straight, lift your leg towards the ceiling, leading with your heel.

Lower to start position, and then lift.

Bring it back to the starting position, not to the ground.

Perform two sets of 10 repetitions, twice a day.

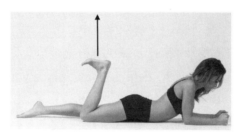

Photo 22: Buttock press

Standing hip extension

Stand upright with good posture, feet shoulder-width apart.

Hold on to a chair, or another fixed surface, for balance.

With your knee straight, extend your leg behind you.

Return to start position and repeat, keeping your balance, without putting your foot on the floor.

Perform two sets of 10 repetitions twice a day.

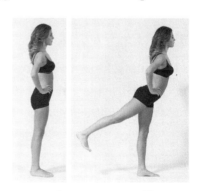

Photos 23A-B: Standing hip extension

Exercises after Surgery on the Chest

The following exercises are to be performed during the second phase of recovery after any procedure on the chest, i.e. breast augmentation, pectoral implants, or liposuction. The purpose of these exercises is to break down adhesions and increase range of motion. Typically start these exercises 3-4 weeks post surgery date.

Scapular retractions

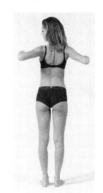

Stand with your arms at your sides, elbows bent to 90 degrees.

Squeeze shoulder blades together as the arms rotate back and out.

Return to start position and repeat.

Perform two sets of 10 repetitions twice a day.

Photo 24: Scapular retractions

Door stretch

Position your elbows below shoulder level.

With your arms at a 90-degree angle, place your hands firmly against the outside of the doorframe.

Step forward, keeping your arms firmly on the door.

Hold for 10 seconds then step back, returning to the original position.

Move your elbows up to higher level, and then repeat.

Perform two sets of 10 repetitions twice a day.

Shoulder retraction

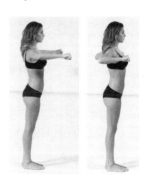

Sit upright in a chair or standing.

Raise arms to shoulder height, out to the side with elbows bent.

Squeeze shoulder blades together, and relax.

Perform two sets of 10 repetitions twice a day.

Photos 25A-B: Shoulder retraction

Chest stretch with arms behind head

Sit with upright posture and hands clasped behind your head.
Squeeze shoulder blades together, and relax.
Perform two sets of 10 repetitions twice a day.

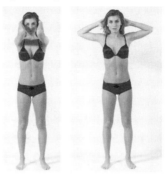

Photos 26A-B: Chest stretch with arms behind head

Exercises after Leg or Thigh Surgery

The following exercises are to be performed during the second phase of recovery after any procedure on the legs, i.e. buttock augmentation or liposuction. The purpose of these exercises is to break down adhesions and increase range of motion. Typically start these exercises 3-4 weeks post surgery date.

Straight leg raise

Lie on your back with your legs straight.

Raise one leg straight up while the other remains on the floor and keep your back flat.

If it is too difficult to keep the bottom leg straight, you may bend it.

Bring your leg back to the starting position.

Perform two sets of 10 repetitions, twice a day. Repeat with the other leg.

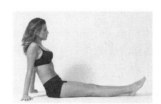
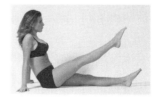

Photos 27A-B: Straight leg raise

Leg raise lying on your side

Lie on your side with your bottom leg bent for stability.

Keep the top leg straight and lift it towards the ceiling.

Do not let your hips roll backwards.

Lower and lift slowly.

Perform two sets of 10 repetitions twice a day. Repeat with the other leg.

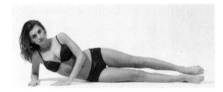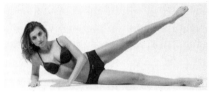

Photos 28A-B: Leg raise lying on your side

Stomach hamstring curl

Laying on your stomach, bend your knee as if to kick your own buttocks.

Return to start position.

Perform two sets of 10 repetitions twice a day. Repeat with the other leg.

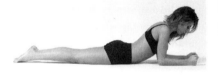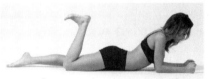

Photos 29A-B: Hamstring curls on stomach

Standing hip extension

Stand upright with good posture, feet shoulder-width apart.

Hold on to a chair or another fixed surface for balance.

With your knee straight, extend your leg behind you.

Return to start position and repeat, without putting your foot on the floor.

Perform two sets of 10 repetitions twice a day. Repeat with the other leg.

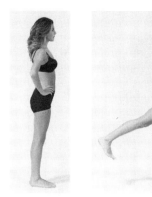

Photos 30A-B: Standing hip extension

Standing hip abduction

Stand upright with good posture, feet shoulder-width apart.

Hold on to a chair or fixed surface for balance.

With your knee straight, kick your leg out to the side.

Return to start position and repeat, without putting your foot on the floor.

Perform two sets of 10 repetitions twice a day. Repeat with the other leg.

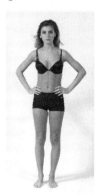
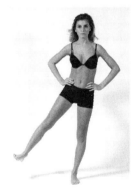

Photos 31A-B: Standing hip abduction

Standing lunges

Stand upright with good posture, feet shoulder-width apart.

Place your hands on your hips for balance if desired.

Step forward, bending your hip and knee to 90 degrees.

Do not let your knee extend past your toes.

Return to start position and repeat.

Perform two sets of 10 repetitions twice a day. Repeat with the other leg.

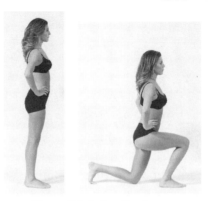

Photos 32A-B: Standing lunges

Standing squats

Stand with your feet shoulder-width apart.

Hold on to a fixed surface.

Squat down, bending your knees, as if you were going to sit on a chair.

Do not let your knees go past your toes.

Return to start position and repeat.

Perform two sets of 10 repetitions twice a day.

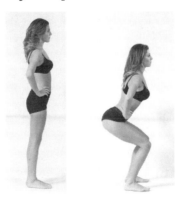

Photos 33A-B: Standing squats

Exercises after Neck Surgery

The following exercises are to be performed during the second phase of recovery after any procedure on the neck, i.e. neck lift, facelift, or liposuction. The purpose of these exercises is to break down adhesions and increase range of motion. Typically start these exercises 3-4 weeks post surgery date.

Neck side bend

Sit upright with good posture, shoulders back.

Gently bend your left ear to your left shoulder, but do not lift your shoulder.

Come back to center then repeat with your right side.

Perform two sets of 10 repetitions twice a day.

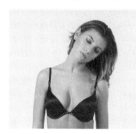 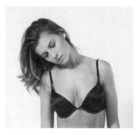

Photos 34A-B: Neck side bend

Neck rotation

Sit upright with good posture, shoulders back.

Gently rotate your head to one side, leading with your nose.

Come back to center then repeat in the opposite direction.

Perform two sets of 10 repetitions twice a day.

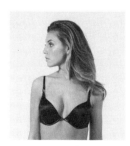 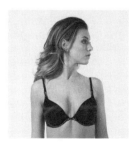

Photos 35A-B: Neck rotation

Neck flexion and extension

Sit upright, shoulders back, with good posture.

Gently extend your head backwards, looking up to the ceiling.

Come back to center, then flex your head forward, bringing your chin to your chest.

Perform two sets of 10 repetitions twice a day.

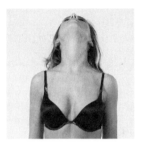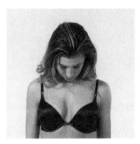

Photos 36A-B: Neck flexion and extension

Chapter 12

How to Improve Your Scar

It is important to know about scar formation and what you can do to prevent your scars from lasting a lifetime. In this chapter I provide you with knowledge about how to improve your scars—one of the final steps in recovery after cosmetic plastic surgery.

By now, you have learned that after any incision is cut into the body, there will be a scar. The way a person's scar develops is difficult to predict because every person's body, and its capability for healing, is different. However, despite the differences in scarring, all scars go through the same process of healing. There are things that you can personally do to promote optimal healing and the appearance of the scar.

The development of scar tissue is the body's natural way to heal an open wound or incision. While dead skin and blood cells are cleaned out, collagen and the growth of new tissue closes and seals the wound in the form of a scab.

The body sends proteins, amino acids, white blood cells, and water to rebuild the area, fight infection, and keep it clean. So, oozing blood and pink or clear liquid is normal in the early stages of healing—your body is just cleaning itself out. As this oozing dries, it forms a scab, which acts as a protective barrier that falls off when the wound is fully healed.

Under the skin surface, a significant amount of work is being done on the scar. At the beginning, the scar will typically be red or pink and tend to look thin. The redness of immature scars is caused by the extra blood supply that your body brings to heal the scar. About six to eight weeks after surgery the scar begins to feel thicker.

Sutures may be removed one to two weeks after your surgery, but the process of wound healing to full scar maturation takes six months to two years. How visible the scar is and how fast it develops depend on many factors, i.e. the size of the wound, how quickly it heals, skin type, age and health of the patient, and how well the wound is treated as it is healing. That last part is key—your healing is dependent on your self-care. You need to do active scar care in order to heal the scar. Luckily, once the wound is healed, there are steps you can take once to assist in flattening, softening, and re-pigmenting the scar.

In the example below, which shows healing after breast implants, the healing of the open area under the patient's right breast should be monitored by her doctor.

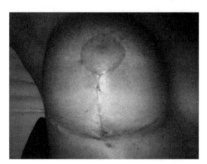 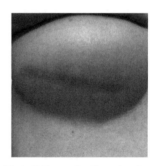

Photo 1: The open area under the patient's right breast (on viewer's left) needs to be monitored by the doctor.

Photo 2: Example of previously infected but now healed incision under the breast

Before we get to self-healing techniques, I have to make sure you know all about scars. Knowing about them will let you better understand your body, your scar, and your healing.

Three Types of Scars

1. Normal Scar

At first, a normal scar may be red but it will usually fade as the wound begins to heal. If the edges of the wound come together neatly and no complications occur, the scar will usually heal as a thin, pale line. Normal scars are typically not painful, although they may be itchy for some months. Typically, a normal scar develops into a flat, thin line that fades over time.

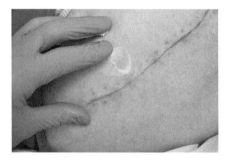

Photo 3: Normal immature scar
(courtesy of shutterstock.com)

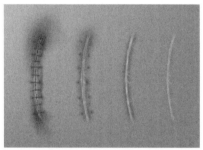

Photo 4: Normal healing scar progression
(courtesy of shutterstock.com)

2. Hypertrophic Scar

A hypertrophic scar may develop as a result of excess collagen and fibrous tissue growth extending into the skin above the scar site. Hypertrophic scars are raised, thick, rough, red, itchy, irregular—but they remain within the limits of the original wound. They are fairly common. When caught early, they respond well to treatment.

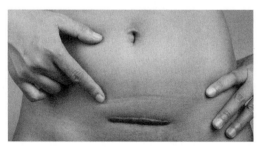

Photo 5: A hypertrophic scar (courtesy of shutterstock.com)

Hypertrophic scarring usually occurs within one to two months of surgery. They have a rapid growth phase for up to six months, then their growth gradually slows down over a few years, eventually leading to a flat scar with no further problems. Hypertrophic scars usually occur following wound infection, wound closure with excess tension, or other traumatic skin injuries. In the majority of cases, hypertrophic scarring develops in places such as the shoulder, neck, sternum, knees and ankles, anterior chest, earlobes, upper arms, and cheeks. Areas generally less prone to hypertrophic scarring include eyelids, cornea, palms, mucous membranes, genitalia, and the soles of the feet.

3. Keloid Scar

A keloid scar is characterized by uncontrolled collagen growth beyond the original injury or trauma site. These scars are the result of an overly aggressive healing process involving the continuous multiplication of fibroblasts (fiber cells) even after the wound is healed closed. Keloids are characterized by thick, puckered, itchy clusters of scar tissue that grow beyond the edges of the wound. Keloids appear as firm, mildly tender, nodular tumors with a shiny surface and sometimes dilated blood vessels called spider veins. Keloids are pink to purple in color and may be accompanied by hyperpigmentation, i.e. darkening of the skin color. The borders of the keloid scar are well-defined but irregular in pattern.

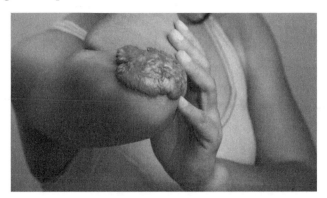

Photo 6: A keloid scar (courtesy of shutterstock.com)

Unlike hypertrophic scars, keloids emerge at least three months or more after the injury. Keloids may develop up to several years after minor injuries. Keloids usually persist for long periods of time, and do not spontaneously stop growing. Due to their severity, they typically require an aggressive treatment plan. Treatments include surgery to remove the scar, steroid injections, or silicone sheets to flatten the scar. Smaller keloids can be treated using cryotherapy—freezing with liquid nitrogen. Keloid formation can be prevented by using pressure treatment or gel pads.

Keloid scars are most common among people with dark skin, and most commonly occur on the earlobes, jaw line, face, and sternum.

Hypertrophic Scars versus Keloids

Here are the differences between the two more severe types of scarring, hypertrophic and keloid scars:

Hypertrophic Scars	Keloid Scars
Regress with time	Grow for years
Remain confined to border of original wound	Extend beyond border of original wound
Arise in any location; common on extensor surfaces	Commonly occur on sternum, shoulders, of joints, upper arms, earlobes, and cheeks
Fewer thick collagen fibers	Thick collagen
Flatten spontaneously over time	Remain elevated more than 4 mm
Appear within one month after surgery	Appear within 3+ months after surgery
Less association with skin pigmentation	More association with darker skin types

Factors That Affect Scarring

Preventing scars means focusing on the factors that you can control. Some forms of prevention are easy, like following the instructions your surgeon gives you, and some are not so simple, like quitting smoking. If you are seriously concerned about scarring, consider discussing the following methods of scar minimization and prevention with your surgeon. Your surgeon may be able to prescribe additional treatments that lower your chances of scarring.

Proper Wound Care

General incision care techniques are essential to healing without scars. Prevent infection by following the instructions given to you by your doctor, and refrain from using ointments and remedies that are not prescribed.

Surgical Technique

Only employ a board-certified/accredited surgeon for your cosmetic surgery. A skilled surgeon will use appropriate and atraumatic sutures for the specific area of your body as well as an appropriate surgical closure to reduce tension on the wound. In other words, having a surgeon who knows what he or she is doing is a key factor in your lifelong healing process.

Postoperative Care

Timely removal of sutures, using dressings and Steri-Strips as support for the scar in the early stages of healing so the scar doesn't open up, use of scar creams and silicone sheets, and cross-friction massage—all of these are important in minimizing scarring.

Exposure to Sunlight

It is very important to avoid exposing your scar to sunlight for one year after your surgery. Sunlight can cause permanent discoloration of your scar. Once the scar is closed, and there are no scabs present, apply daily SPF of 50. SPF lotion over scars is key!

Size and Depth of Your Incision

The deeper and longer the incision, the longer the healing process will take and the greater the opportunity for scarring. A larger incision may also be exposed to more stress as you move, which can cause slower healing.

Location of the Scar

Incisions in the armpit, under the knee or elbow, or anywhere that crosses a joint will more likely scar than one that does not. Areas that bend or move a lot are the most susceptible to the scar stretching, i.e. knee, shoulder, and back. For example, if a scar crosses the knee joint and you aggressively bend your knee too far, too quickly, it can cause the scar to be larger.

Direction of the Scar

The direction of the scar also plays a large role in how it appears. Scars that are aligned with natural relaxed skin creases and lines will remain thinner and less noticeable than scars that travel across the skin lines. Scars that can be camouflaged on the face, i.e. along the eyebrow or side of the nose, will be less noticeable.

Stress on Your Incision

Lifting, bending, or doing anything that stretches or puts tension on your incision can pull the incision apart, delay healing, and will often make the wound larger. Making the wound larger increases the size of your scar.

Dehiscence of the Wound

Dehiscence means that the incision separates and opens up. This can be caused by any of the stresses listed above as well as trauma, removal of sutures too soon, and swelling which increases tension on the wound.

Skin Tone

Research has shown that certain skin tones are more likely to scar than others. Those who are very fair, especially redheads, tend to scar more than those with olive complexions. Darker skin tones are more likely to form hypertrophic and keloid scars.

Genetics

If you have a family tendency to scar badly, you are likely to scar badly. Genetics play a huge role in all aspects of healing.

Age

As a person gets older, skin loses elasticity and becomes thinner. This is because collagen, which makes your skin elastic, changes as you age, and the fat layer under your skin becomes thinner.

Skin Tightness

Patients with saggy skin and decreased elasticity, whether due to age or significant weight loss, will develop less scar tissue because there is reduced tension when closing the skin together after surgery. If you have taut, tight skin, you will be more likely to develop noticeable scars because of the skin tension that occurs during the suturing process.

Nutrition

Poor nutrition impairs healing. Poor healing means a bigger scar. Making sure there is a good amount of protein and vitamins in your diet helps promote healing.

Tobacco Use

Smoking and other forms of tobacco and nicotine use increase your risk for scars and slow healing time. Smoking and these allied habits also put a patient at risk for complications during surgery and postoperatively.

Alcohol

Alcohol dehydrates both the body and skin. This decreases your overall state of health and interferes with scar healing.

Hydration

Dehydration is the result of not taking in enough water and fluids. Dehydration interferes with scar healing. Drink plenty of water!

Weight

Being overweight puts you at greater risk for scarring because the fat under your skin can put more tension on the closing of the incision closing during surgery.

Rest

Exhaustion and lack of sleep can impair wound healing. The body naturally heals itself during sleep—so make sure to get plenty of rest.

Pre-existing Medical Conditions

Medical conditions, i.e. diabetes mellitus or poor circulation, can slow scar healing. Any medical condition you have should be well-controlled before surgery to ensure the best recovery.

Infection

If your incision becomes infected, it is important to identify the signs of infection as soon as possible and contact your physician immediately. An infection can seriously impair healing and can contribute to scarring.

Signs and Symptoms of an Infected Surgical Incision

Fever

A fever greater than 100.4 degrees Fahrenheit, accompanied by chills.

Hot Incision

An infected incision may feel hot to the touch because the body sends infection fighting blood cells to the incision site.

Swelling or Hardening of the Incision

The incision itself may appear swollen, puffy, and begin to harden as the tissue underneath becomes inflamed.

Redness

An incision that becomes red, or begins to have red streaks radiating from it and the surrounding skin, may be infected.

Pain

As you heal, your pain should slowly and steadily diminish. If for no apparent reason, your pain at the surgery site increases, you may be developing an infection in the wound.

Fatigue

When recovering from surgery it is common to feel exhausted, but it is typical to feel better each day. If you have a sudden onset of severe fatigue, days after surgery, it might be a sign of infection.

Open Area

If the incision site separates, this could cause an infection or be a sign of an infection. If there is pus coming out of the open incision, it is definitely infected. This is called dehiscence of the incision.

Incision Growing in Size

A change in the size of the incision—getting longer or spreading to the sides—is a sign of an infection.

Severe Bleeding

Bleeding so excessive that it soaks through the dressing is bad news. Call your doctor.

Pus Draining from the Incision

Foul-smelling drainage or pus that ranges in color from blood-tinged to green, white, or yellow. The infected drainage may also be thick and, in rare instances, chunky.

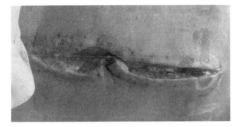

Photo 7: An infected incision which was red, hot, and draining foul-smelling yellow pus from an open area (dehiscence). (courtesy of shutterstock.com)

Incision Care after Surgery to Promote Good Scar Healing

Right after surgery, sutures are used to hold the edges of the skin together. Until the epidermis—the top layer of skin—heals, there may be some scabs present. If your incision is covered with butterfly closures, i.e. Steri-Strips, do not remove them. Butterfly closures should be allowed to fall off naturally. If the incision is open to air and you see scabs, doctors commonly recommend using topical antibiotic cream such as Bacitracin or Polysporin, for the first 10 to 14 days after surgery to protect the healing tissue and to keep the scabs from getting too hard. You should never pick the scabs off—they should be allowed to fall off naturally. Picking at scabs is very likely to increase scarring as well as slow healing.

General Directions for Incision Care

Please follow any specific instructions your doctor or nurse may give you. The following are general instructions based on my own personal experience and my experience with patients:

- Wash your hands before caring for your incision.
- Do not apply any creams, salves, ointments, or powders unless you have been told to do so.
- You may take a shower. Remove the dressing before your shower. After your shower, pat the incision site dry with a clean towel and put on a new dressing.
- Do not take a tub bath until your doctor says it's okay.
- When you are not in the shower, keep the incision site as clean and dry as possible, i.e. if the dressing is on your hand or arm, do not wash dishes.
- Do not poke, scratch, or rub your incision.
- Your incision may have some clear or slightly bloody. This is normal as long as the incision continues to drain less each day.

- Do not pull, cut, or interfere with any sutures (stitches) the surgeon has made. The doctor will remove all sutures when indicated. This usually happens at the one or two week post-op visit.
- Keep your Steri-Strips™ on until they fall off naturally.
- It is okay for butterfly closures, i.e. Steri-Strips™, to get wet, just pat them dry after showering. Just try not to soak them!
- Do not shower if you still have drains in your wound area.
- After the drain(s) are removed, you must wait 48 hours before showering.
- Keep incisions clean and inspect daily for signs of infection.

Changing the Dressing over an Incision

- Wash your hands before starting the dressing change.
- Remove the old dressing by touching only the edges. Throw away the old dressing in the garbage.
- Wash your hands again.
- Open a sterile dressing package by holding the upper two edges of the package and pulling sideways, rather than tearing the package open.
- Keep the new dressing inside the sterile package until you are ready to put it over your incision.
- Touch only the edges of the new dressing. Do not touch any part of the dressing that will be on the incision.
- It is best to use a non-stick dressing, i.e. a Telfa pad.
- Tape all sides of the dressing securely.
- Wash your hands after you have finished applying the new dressing.
- If there is a drainage tube, be sure to cover this area with the dressing.
- Follow any special instructions your doctor or nurse has given to you.

How to Treat an Infected Incision

Oral Antibiotics

If you are not on antibiotics already, your doctor may prescribe one for you.

Clean the Incision

Your doctor may give you a specific soap or cleanser to wash out the infected incision.

Wet sterile bandages may be placed inside the wound and left to dry. Other wet or dry dressings may also be used.

Topical Cream

Your doctor may prescribe a topical cream or ointment to treat the infected incision. This may or may not be an antibiotic. Silvadene is a commonly used non-antibiotic prescription cream that makes skin conditions unfavorable for the growth of bacteria. It is also used as a burn cream.

Pain Relief

Your doctor may recommend that you take a medication containing either an NSAID or acetaminophen to reduce pain or fever.

How to Treat a Normal Scar

Here are 14 different ways you can best heal your scar. Always consult with your doctor before starting any treatment plan.

Pressure Therapy

Pressure therapy is provided by a pressure appliance that is worn over the area of the scar, i.e. a compression garment or pressure dressing. Pressure therapy has been the favorite type of conservative treatment for both hypertrophic scars and keloids scars since the 1970s. The aim of pressure therapy is to flatten and soften scars.

A compression garment causes faster wound healing, reduces risk of complications, controls swelling, increases blood flow to the wound, and supports the scar, skin, and underlying muscle and fat. The mechanism of action of pressure therapy is not fully understood. Some research suggests that because the compression garment limits the supply of blood, oxygen, and nutrients to the scar tissue, the formation of collagen is decreased and more unnecessary fiber cells die.

Pressure dressings are usually used under the supervision of a specialist. They are usually made from a stretchy, elastic material. They are worn over the scar 24 hours a day for six to 12 months. They can also be used over a long period of time in combination with silicone gel sheeting to improve the appearance of scars.

Recommendations for the amount of pressure and wearing schedule is 15–40 mm Hg for at least 23 hours and/or one day for more than six months while the scar's healing process is still active. Two factors that negatively affect pressure therapy are inability to appropriately fit the garment to the wounded area and patient discomfort. These factors may affect compliance with wearing these garments or dressings.

Silicone Sheets

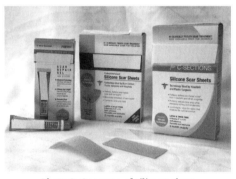

Photo 8: One type of silicone sheet

Topical silicone gel sheeting has been a well-established treatment for management of scars since its introduction in the early 1980s. Following the National Institute of Health's studies on the material in 2002, many companies have introduced versions of thin silicone sheeting for postoperative care after plastic surgery. Similar in appearance to plastic wrap, the material is applied to your incisions once they've reached adequate maturity—no open areas on the incision, the scabs have naturally fallen off, and there is no drainage.

The benefits of silicone sheets include the non-stick quality, the ability to protect the incision during dressing changes, and the creation of an environment that retains water and keeps out harmful chemical, bacterial, and particulate material out of the body. Its therapeutic effects on hypertrophic scars have been well-researched, and it is clear that silicone gel sheets help flatten hypertrophic and keloid scars.

Silicone sheets should be worn for at least 12 hours a day. However, they are most effective if worn 24 hours a day for at least three months.

Silicone sheets can be cut to fit the incision area, which helps you get more out of your supply of silicone sheets and is more comfortable to wear.

Some examples of silicone sheet products

Biodermis®

ScarAway®

Scar Fx®

Dermatix®

Silicone Gel

Some surgical incisions on complex dimensional areas of the body, i.e. the joints or the face, are hard to dress with a flat sheeting material. Silicone gel was created as an alternative way to address this issue.

This version of silicone treatment binds with the outermost layer of your skin for the same healing benefits of silicone sheeting, plus it has the advantage of easy application anywhere on the body. Certain silicone gel treatments come with added

SPF ingredient that protects the newly formed skin of the scar from pigmentation irregularities that can develop if the scar is left unshielded and exposed to direct sunlight.

Some examples of silicone gel products

> Bio Corenum®
>
> NewGel®
>
> Scar Fade Arbonne®
>
> Scarguard®

Some examples of new combination treatments

> Implantech makes the Gelzone® Wrap, which combines both silicone scar therapy with gentle compression.
>
> Embrace® combines silicone sheeting with active tension release over the scar.

Topical Scar Cream

Over-the-counter scar therapies can promote healing by causing a nice seal over a scar. Flavonoids are plant extracts that help wound healing and blood vessel health. They are found in well-known topical scar creams. Recent research has shown that these creams inhibit fibroblast proliferation and collagen production, and cause fibroblasts in hypertrophic and keloid scars to contract. Some research suggests that a skin moisturizer containing alpha-hydroxy acids promotes skin health and scar fading. Speak with your doctor about choosing the best option for you.

Some examples of topical creams

> Mederma Advance®
>
> ScarGuard MD®
>
> Scarlight MD®
>
> Strataderm®

Keeping the scar moisturized is also an important part of the healing process. This also helps the healing process by increasing the skin's collagen production, which is essential to healing. Choose a lotion without perfume or dye.

Some examples of moisturizing lotions

Eucerin®

Lubriderm®

Nivea®

Cetaphil®

Natural Topical Remedies

These are natural products you can use to help heal your scar.

Raw honey

One of the traditional methods to promote healing is to apply honey to your wound. Honey can be used directly on the scar while it is still healing because the enzymes in the honey are active as both an antiseptic and a healing agent. In 2006, a review of over twenty clinical trials of honey that involved over 2,000 patients showed that honey stimulated the growth of new tissue as well as having anti-inflammatory and anti-bacterial properties.

St. John's wort (hypericum)

Hypericum stimulates collagen growth and helps scar tissue to form in a way leading to a quick and healthy recovery. One study found that those treated with St. John's wort within 24 hours after surgery had less itching, less discomfort, faster healing times, less skin discoloration, and flatter and more even scars.

Shea and cocoa butters

Shea and cocoa butters are each thick, waxy, natural oils that come from the seeds of a tree. Humans have used both of them for centuries as a natural moisturizer for dry and cracked skin. It is recommended to use it as the pure oil. Rub it into the newly formed scar several times a day. If you are unable to obtain these natural oils in their pure form, they are also available in creams, lotions, and ointments.

Aloe vera

The use of aloe vera can be traced back 6,000 years to ancient Egypt where it was known as the plant of immortality. Aloe vera's anti-inflammatory and moisturizing properties may help reduce the swelling and redness of the scar. It has the ability to penetrate deeply into the skin, repair damaged cells, protect new cells, and increase the amount of collagen produced. Aloe vera has also been highly regarded as a treatment for burns.

Vitamin E

For years topical vitamin E has been a common remedy recommended by doctors, yet research has not clearly supported its reported ability to reduce scars. Although it has not been proven to directly reduce scarring when topically applied to the area, it may help the body through the healing process if taken orally as a daily supplement. Vitamin E is essential to the body as a powerful antioxidant that is thought to slow aging, protect arteries, reduce bad cholesterol, and help combat heart disease.

Surgical Revision

If you've recently had surgery that left you with scars, it is best to wait at least one year before making a decision about surgical scar treatment. Many scars fade and become less noticeable over time. Surgical removal remains the traditional treatment for keloids and hypertrophic scars.

Depending on your particular situation, there may be many options to treat deeper scars, including skin grafts, excision (surgical removal), dermabrasion, and laser surgery. If your scarring impairs function, surgery can help address the functional problems.

One negative to think about is the fact that surgically removing the scar can result in a longer or bigger scar than the original hypertrophic scar or keloid.

Here is a list of surgical procedures that can be performed to reduce scars:

Subcision

This technique is used to break the bands of scar under the skin.

Dermaroller or microneedling

This is a minimally invasive skin-rejuvenation procedure that uses a device that contains many fine needles. This is ideal for medium-level scars. Four to six sessions are required. The downtime is minimal and usually limited to redness and swelling for a few hours. It is most often used for treating acne scars.

Z-plasty and related tissue-rearrangement techniques

Z-plasty is a plastic surgery technique used to reorient a scar to make it less noticeable. The scar is re-oriented by cutting the skin around the scar into small triangular flaps. Although the technique your doctor chooses will depend on the shape of the scar, these flaps usually follow a "Z" shape. The flaps are repositioned to follow the natural lines and creases of the skin. Z-plasty can also help relieve the pressure of contracture scars.

Dermabrasion

Dermabrasion is a process that removes the top layer of skin, smoothing out surface irregularities such as deep lines or scars.

After the target area is injected with anesthetic, the desired amount of skin is removed by gentle sanding with a rotating wire brush or a diamond wheel.

Tissue expansion

Tissue expansion is a technique used by plastic surgeons to cause the body to grow additional skin. In this procedure, a small balloon is inserted under a patch of healthy skin near a scar. Saline (salt) solution is injected into the balloon to stretch the skin. The balloon remains in the body for a few weeks or months, and then is removed after the skin has been adequately stretched. The scar is then surgically excised (removed), and the newly stretched skin is pulled over the previously scarred area and sutured closed.

Collagen injections

Collagen is the main natural structural protein found in animals, including humans. Collagen injections are used to raise or fill in sunken scars. The results of collagen injections are immediate but not permanent. The body slowly absorbs the collagen, so eventually the scars will have to be refilled.

Skin grafting

In this procedure, doctors take skin from a healthy part of the body and transplant it to the injured area. This technique is commonly used on people who have been severely burned. Although a scar will also form in the area where the graft came from, a skin graft can greatly restore function in a severely scarred area. Since the result may not be cosmetically pleasing, skin grafting is often performed out of necessity rather than for cosmetic enhancement.

Vascular laser

A vascular laser works by shrinking the blood vessels that feed the scar, thus improving the coloration of red scars. This treatment is performed without anesthetic and the average treatment time is 15 minutes. On average, one to three sessions are needed to achieve optimal results.

Laser Treatment of Keloids

Laser treatment of keloids was introduced in the mid-1980s. Resurfacing skin by using a laser can be a very effective way to treat scarring. Lasers remove the topmost layers of skin, allowing new, smooth skin to form. A pattern of pin-sized holes is burned through the dermal and epidermal layers of the skin, stimulating healing of those layers, which are supported by healthy surrounding tissue.

The whole skin surface in the area is treated during the course of several sessions. And some color lasers can effectively treat the abnormal red pigmentation of hypertrophic and keloid scars.

The two types of lasers used for reducing the uneven surface of scars are the CO_2 (carbon dioxide) laser and the Er:YAG (erbium-doped yttrium aluminum garnet) laser. The CO_2 laser is typically used for deeper scars, while the Er:YAG laser is used for superficial scars and deeper skin tones. Research has shown very encouraging results in treating young hypertrophic scars and keloids using a 585-nanometer pulsed-dye laser (PDL).

Two to six treatments may be necessary to successfully improve scar factors including scar color, height, pliability, and texture. Side effects of laser treatment include discoloration and blistering. The most common adverse side effect is skin discoloration to a purple hue, which fortunately usually goes away after seven to 10 days.

Corticosteroid Injections

Corticosteroid injections are used to treat some keloid and hypertrophic scars. These injections can also help reduce the itching and/or pain associated with these scars. This treatment cannot remove scars, but it can improve their appearance and help flatten and reduce the redness of hypertrophic and keloid scars.

Multiple small injections are made into the scar to reduce any swelling due to inflammation and to flatten the scar. Corticosteroids are applied to or injected into the scar to break down collagen in the skin. If you are prone to forming keloid scars, talk to your surgeon about having a steroid injection to prevent the formation of another keloid.

Depending on the type of scar, these may need to be repeated. Usually injections are given on three occasions at intervals of four to six weeks to assess your body's response. If the scar is improving, sometimes treatment may continue for several months.

Side effects include dermal atrophy and increased sensitivity and pain at the site of injection. Local anesthetic can be used to address pain at the injection site.

Cryotherapy

Cryotherapy refers to a treatment in which lesions on the surface of the skin are frozen. Cryotherapy has been used alone as well as along with other forms of treatment for excessive scars. Specifically, the combination of cryotherapy with injections seems to show marked improvement of hypertrophic scars and keloids, but research has shown that the benefits of cryotherapy are limited to the management of small scars. Several weeks between sessions are usually required for postoperative healing and there are some common side effects, including permanent hypo- and hyperpigmentation, moderate skin atrophy, blistering, and postoperative pain.

Diet and Nutrition

Eat a balanced, vitamin-enriched diet with an emphasis on protein. Your cells use the amino acids found in protein as building blocks to produce new cells to promote scar healing.

Chicken, pork, fish, seafood, beef, dairy, and soy are all good sources of protein. Eat plenty of fresh fruits and vegetables. Cut down on calories, fatty foods, and starchy carbs. The more nutritional and antioxidant value your food has, the better your body can heal.

Drink plenty of fresh, clean water. Filtered water is optimal.

Coffee and other caffeinated beverages, alcohol, and sodas will not help.

One glass of red wine is rich in antioxidants and okay to drink once a day, but more than that will hurt more than help.

Green tea and herbal tea have a lot of beneficial health-giving properties and antioxidants.

While your wound is healing, try to avoid caffeinated beverages because caffeine dehydrates the body. Nothing is better for your body's healing than plenty of water.

Taking vitamins is just as necessary for the best healing as watching what you eat. Vitamin C is an important supplement to take to support the healing process. Vitamin C helps our bodies produce collagen which heals our wounds. Without vitamin C, our bodies can't produce collagen and cannot heal as well—this is why it's especially important to take Vitamin C both before and after surgery. Aim for 500 mg twice a day until the incision is completely healed.

Avoid Exposure to Direct Sunlight

Avoid exposing the scar to sunlight for one year. Use sunblock and proper attire to keep the incision covered. While the scar is still immature and red, it is not recommended to use sun block on the scar. If you get a tan on an immature scar, the pigment will get trapped and make the scar more visible for the rest of your life.

Avoid and Treat Blistering

Blistering on the skin surrounding the scar is caused by reduced elasticity in dressing and increased edema dermatitis (blisters caused by swelling).

It is important that you use non-adhesive or low-adhesive tape instead of regular tape. While you may think it's easier to use the Scotch tape you have lying around your house, you will only make your scar worse. Adhesive dressing tape usually costs less than $10 a roll. It's affordable and better for your healing in the long run—so use it!

Makeup

Cosmetic camouflage makeup is specially designed for covering up scars, not treating them. You can buy it online or over the counter at makeup counters and pharmacies. Cosmetic camouflage can be particularly useful for facial scars because it can temporarily but quickly hide the scar.

Some cosmetic camouflage makeup is waterproof and can stay in place for two to three days—nice because you don't have to continually reapply it every morning.

It is important to undergo color testing in order to get the makeup that is best suited for your skin tone and which will cover your scars most effectively. However, finding the correct color can be a lengthy process, sometimes taking over an hour, so I recommend going to the pharmacy when you have enough time to pick out the perfect camouflage color, and make sure you have makeup testing performed by a qualified makeup color tester. Makeup prices can range from about $18 to $70 for a half-ounce jar or tube.

Some examples of camouflage makeup products

Coverderm®

Dermablend®

Dermaflage®

Smart Cover®

Massage Can Make a Scar Smaller

Massage is commonly used on post-surgical incisions to help make the scar smaller, flatter, and less visible.

Be sure to check with your doctor or physical therapist to ensure that proper healing has taken place before starting scar tissue massage and that scar tissue massage is appropriate. Massaging a scar that is not fully healed can cause damage to the developing scar tissue. This can delay healing and possibly also create more scarring.

In general, the scar must be fully closed with no scabbing present and with all staples and sutures removed before beginning scar massage. Massaging the incision area and the surrounding tissue may even out any bumps or lumps that remain after the healing process.

Cross-Friction Massage

Cross-friction massage is sometimes called trans-friction massage. This technique helps to remodel the scar and ensures that the collagen fibers of the scar are aligned properly. Another purpose of cross-friction massage is to maintain mobility within the soft tissue structures of ligaments, tendons, and muscles and prevent other scars from forming.

This massage is deep and must be applied perpendicular to the scar. This means that you are massaging across the scar— not along the scar. Detailed instructions for performing cross-friction massage are given below.

Benefits of cross-friction massage

Decreased inflammation

Breakdown of scar tissue, which restores the flow of lymph fluid

Increased capillary proliferation, which facilitates healing

Desensitized scar

Rehydrated and softened scar tissue

Promotes collagen remodeling by applying pressure to scar

Helps to decrease itching

Improves scar flexibility

Flattens the scar

When to start performing cross-friction massage

Start one week after removal of sutures, but only if the wound is fully healed. This usually means starting two to three weeks after surgery.

For best results, perform cross-friction massage two to three times a day for five to 10 minutes at a time and for at least three months.

Short but regular episodes of firm-pressure massage to the scar stimulate the body to more efficiently mature the scar. This avoids excess tissue firmness and swelling while more quickly fading the pink color of the scar.

When to stop performing cross-friction massage

Stop the massage process and contact your doctor if you experience any of the following:

Redness

Bleeding

Scar feels warmer than the skin around it

Scar is no longer closed—open areas appear

More pain than usual at the site of the scar

Method for Cross-Friction Massage

A small amount of moisturizing ointment should be used during cross-friction massage to keep the tissue lubricated and avoid irritation. The moisturizer should be hypoallergenic, containing no dyes or perfumes.

Start with gentle pressure, and then begin to add pressure as tolerated. Massage must be firm to be effective—as soon as you remove the pressure of your hand, the scar must blanch (white).

Use one or two fingers to massage your scar in a direction that is perpendicular to the line of the scar. Use the pads or soft tips of your fingers to massage the scar and tissue around the scar.

Starting at one end of the scar, massage in one spot for about a minute. Then gradually move the area of massage along the scar in small steps so you finally have massaged the entire length of the scar area.

It is normal for cross-friction massage to hurt—in fact, it almost always hurts. If it doesn't hurt at all, you are probably in the wrong spot or you are not applying enough pressure.

Techniques for Cross-Friction Massage

Massage in all three directions—circles, vertical, and horizontal.

Circles

Using two fingers make small circles over the length of the scar and the skin surrounding it.

Vertical

Using two fingers massage the scar up-and-down.

Horizontal

Using two fingers massage the scar from side to side.

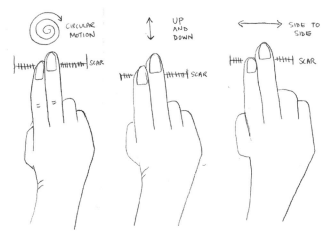

Photo 9: The three techniques for cross-friction massage

Alternative Massage Therapy

If you find that performing massage using your hands is too difficult, you can use a therapy tool to assist you. A mini-vibrator has a rubber tip and is battery-powered to massage your scar. You can buy one online or contact a medical supply distributor. One example is a mini-vibrator produced by North Coast Medical which costs about $40.

Section Four

Surgery-Specific Information

Chapter 13
General Instructions for Care after Cosmetic Surgery

Activity

Get plenty of rest after surgery.

When getting out of bed, sit up carefully and then stand slowly to prevent fainting.

Start walking as soon as possible! Walking helps to reduce swelling and lowers the chance of blood clots.

Do not overexert yourself.

No lifting greater than five pounds, i.e. a gallon of milk, for at least one to two weeks—and longer for certain specific surgeries.

Limit vigorous physical activity for several weeks. Examples include heavy housework, sex, bending, or any activity that raises your blood pressure.

If you are not sure whether it is okay to do an activity, it's best to ask your doctor rather than taking a risk.

Do not drive until you are no longer taking pain medication.

Wear your garment as prescribed.

Wear compression stockings.

Do specific exercises as described in previous chapters.

Generally, avoid having sex for two weeks, and then have careful sex for two weeks.

Skin Care

Bathing

When showering, use a hypoallergenic soap, i.e. Dial.

Ice

Apply ice to the surgery area as often as possible for three to five days immediately after surgery to decrease swelling. Apply for 30 minutes on and 30 minutes off as a recommended schedule. Use a sheet between your skin and the ice to avoid frostbite.

Antibiotic Cream or Ointment

Apply on incisions to speed up healing. Only use Bacitracin. I do not recommend Neosporin because it may cause increased reddening of the incision.

Hydrocortisone Cream or Ointment

Rub it gently on the skin next to your incision. This will help stop itching. Do not use on incisions or areas that are open.

Sun

Avoid exposing scars to sun for at least 12 months.

Sun block

You should avoid exposure to sunlight while healing, but if you can't avoid being in the sun always wear sunscreen—SPF 50 or greater.

Good Nutrition

Fluids are very important following surgery! Drink plenty of water. Stick to non-carbonated, non-alcoholic, caffeine-free beverages, including fruit juices, milk, and yogurt drinks. You must consume at least eight ounces of fluid every two hours. Stick with soft, bland, nutritious food for the first 24 hours. See Chapter 3 for more about diet and nutrition.

Incision Care

Common Items for Incision Care

1. Non-stick pads

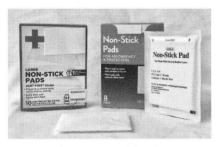

Photo 1: Non-stick pads

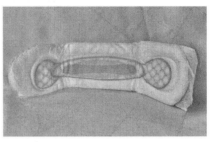

Photo 2: In a pinch - maxi pads can be used over incision sites

2. Bacitracin ointment

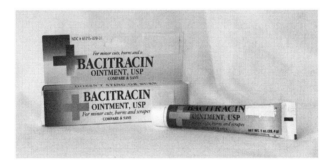

Photo 3: Bacitracin ointment (packaging and manufacturer may vary)

3. Medical paper tape

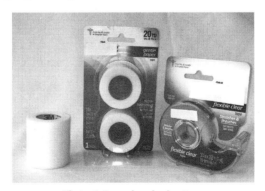

Photo 4: Paper bandaging tape

4. Butterfly closures

These are often called Steri-Strips or adhesive strips.

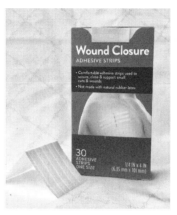

Photo 5: Adhesive strips, one form of butterfly closure

5. Alcohol wipes

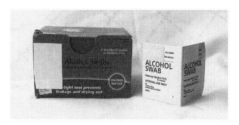

Photo 6: Alcohol wipes

General Directions for Incision Care

Wash your hands before caring for your incision.

Do not apply any creams, salves, ointments, or powders unless you have been told to.

You may take a shower. Remove the dressing before your shower.

After your shower, pat the incision site dry with a clean towel. Put on a new dressing.

Do not take a tub bath until your doctor says it's okay.

When you are not in the shower, keep the incision site as clean and dry as possible. For example, if the dressing is on your hand or arm, do not wash dishes.

Do not poke, scratch, or rub your incision.

Your incision may have drainage that is clear or slightly bloody. This is normal. Expect that the incision should drain less each day.

Keep butterfly closures on and let them fall off naturally.

It's okay to get butterfly closures wet when you shower—just pat them dry after showering.

Do not shower if you still have drains. No tub soaking until sutures or drains are removed.

If a drainage tubes has been placed, you may shower 48 hours after they are removed.

Fluid in your drain is measured in ccs (cubic centimeters) or mls (milliliters). A "cc" and a "ml" are the same volume.

Keep incisions clean and check them daily for signs of infection.

Changing the Dressing over an Incision

Wash your hands before starting the dressing change.

Remove the old dressing by touching only the edges. Throw away the old dressing in the garbage.

Wash your hands again.

Apply Bacitracin

Open a sterile dressing package by holding the upper two edges of the package and pull sideways rather than tearing the package open.

Keep the new dressing inside the sterile package until you are ready to put it over your incision.

Touch only the edges of the new dressing. Do not touch any part of the dressing that will be on the incision.

Use a non-stick dressing pad, i.e. Telfa pad.

Tape all sides of the dressing securely.

Wash your hands when the new dressing is on.

If there is a drainage tube, be sure to cover it with the dressing.

Follow any special instructions your doctor or nurse gives you.

Flying after Surgery

It is recommended that you *do not* fly for at least *two weeks* after surgery.

Even though that is the official recommendation, I suggest to patients that they not fly for at least *one month* after surgery. You do not know how your body is going to react or heal—it's best to stay close to your doctor.

If you cannot avoid flying then do the following:

Take one aspirin on the day of the flight after getting your doctor's approval.

Do ankle pumps every hour.

Drink one eight-ounce bottle of water per hour on the flight

Walk in the plane's aisle once an hour.

Don't use caffeine the day of the flight.

Don't use alcohol the day of the flight.

Don't sit with your legs crossed.

Chapter 14
Care of the Face after Surgery

These are general recommendations—speak to your doctor about specific recommendations they may have regarding your procedure

Cheek Implant

You should be able to return to work and your other normal activities within a week, depending on the intensity of your job.

You should rest in a face-up position at a 45-degree angle for at least one week.

Stitches are removed in five to 10 days. Sutures placed inside the mouth will dissolve in a similar period of time.

You may be restricted to a soft diet for up to 10 days.

After four to six weeks, vigorous physical activity can be resumed.

Occasionally cheek implants must be held temporarily in place using *bolsters*—small pads sutured over the cheek implant site. If used, these bolsters are removed in about six to seven days.

During the first week after placement of your implant, it is important that you avoid bumping or traumatizing the implant while it is becoming fixed in place. Once the body has begun incorporating the implant in a layer of scar tissue, dislodging the implant becomes much more difficult.

Avoid sleeping on your stomach or side, as this will put pressure on the implant.

Sleep with your head elevated on at least two pillows.

Ear Surgery (Otoplasty)

Avoid bending, lifting, pulling, pushing, straining, and aerobic activities for three weeks.

Adults can go back to work approximately one week after surgery, depending upon their occupation.

Avoid any activity in which the ear might be bent for approximately a month.

Some people may resume moderate exercise after three weeks—check with your doctor. Strenuous activity may be resumed as soon as one to two months—or no sooner than eight to nine months. Check with your doctor to find out when you can safely resume strenuous activity.

Sleep on your back. Avoid sleeping on the operated ear.

Sleep with your head elevated for at least two weeks.

Wear turban-style dressings and bandages for three to four days. After that, wear a clean headband at night for three to six weeks.

You may shampoo your hair one week after surgery, unless your doctor tells you otherwise.

Some swelling and bruising may last for 10 to 14 days.

Tenderness could last for up to three months.

Both ears will not match perfectly, as perfect symmetry of ears is unlikely and unnatural.

All sutures/stitches are removed, or will dissolve, one to two weeks after surgery.

Incisions are behind the ear. Your doctor may have you apply antibiotic ointment with a Q-tip 1-2 times a day.

No pull-over clothing, i.e. t-shirts, sweatshirts, crew-neck sweaters, for two weeks.

Avoid chewing hard or tough foods for two weeks.

Eyelid Surgery (Blepharoplasty)

Occasionally the eyes are bandaged for the first night.

Avoid activities that raise your blood pressure, including bending, lifting, and rigorous sports.

Keep activities to a minimum for three to five days.

Avoid strenuous activities for two to three weeks.

Read or watch television after two to three days.

Return to work in 10 to 14 days.

Your hair can be shampooed any time after surgery.

Wait at least two weeks before wearing contact lenses.

For the first few weeks, you may experience excessive tearing, sensitivity to light, and double or blurred vision.

You will be sensitive to sunlight, wind, and other irritants for several weeks, so wear sunglasses and a special sun block made for eyelids.

Expect temporary eyelid swelling, tightness, bruising, dryness, burning, and itching.

You may have gummy eyes—a sticky eye discharge—for approximately one week.

Your physician may recommend Natural Tears or Lacri-Lube ophthalmic ointment as part of your postoperative care. These products are available without prescription.

Tobradex eye drops may be prescribed to decreases inflammation.

Sutures will usually be removed in five to seven days.

You may have difficulty closing your eyes when you sleep.

Sleep with your head elevated.

Avoid sleeping on your stomach.

A bag of frozen peas may best conform to the area, instead of an ice pack.

Facelift (Rhytidectomy) or Neck Lift

No strenuous activities for at least two weeks, i.e. sex or heavy housework.

Do not play sports, i.e. tennis, golf, swimming, running, yoga, or dance, or perform heavy yard work for four to six weeks after surgery.

Avoid vigorous workouts for four to six weeks after surgery.

Walking and mild stretching are fine. Light cardio activity, i.e. walking moderate distances outside or light treadmill/ stationary bike, may be resumed three weeks after surgery if your doctor approves.

Do not lift anything over 10 pounds, i.e. small children, groceries, and suitcases, for four to six weeks after surgery.

Return to work in two to three weeks.

Sleep with head on two pillows to reduce swelling.

Do not sleep on your stomach.

Bruising and swelling around the eyes is common. Ice compresses or a bag of frozen peas or corn may be applied to the eyes to help reduce swelling after your operation. Place a moist cloth or gauze over each eye, then place the cool pack over it. Do not put ice directly on your eyelids.

Leave the cool pack on the eyes for 20–30 minutes, and then remove it for ten minutes. Repeat this as tolerated for the first 24 hours after surgery.

Most of the noticeable swelling and bruising will decrease during the first three to four weeks after surgery.

Most people look presentable to the public about three to four weeks after surgery, although, you may still have residual bruising requiring cover-up makeup. It may take two to three months for all signs of surgery—swelling, bruising, and redness— to completely resolve.

Do not use hair dye or permanent-wave solution until approved by your surgeon.

Hair is generally shampooed on the second or third postoperative day. The area of sutures must be washed gently but thoroughly each time.

Do not set hair-dryer temperature on hot, as you may not have sensation in operated areas and thus may not know that you are getting burned.

You may use makeup after the sutures are removed. New facial makeup can be used to cover up bruising, but not on the incisions. Using a new package of makeup that has not previously been opened is recommended because previously opened or used makeup may not be completely clean and thus may cause infection. It is important to gently remove all makeup.

Wear a facial compression sling for compression and support.

You may experience tightness in your neck and difficulty turning your neck side to side for one to two months.

Your skin may feel dry and rough for several months.

Men will have a need to shave behind their ears because beard-growing skin was repositioned there.

Sutures are usually removed from in front of the ear in three to five days. Any remaining sutures and metal clips, if used, are usually removed in one to two weeks.

Drains are usually removed one to three days after surgery. Some bloody drainage into the bulb of the drain is normal. Excessive drainage, such as more than 50 cc/ml per eight-hour period is abnormal. You should report this to your doctor promptly.

If you have drainage tubes, you may not shower until 48 hours after they are removed.

You may bathe 48 hours after surgery. Avoid steam baths and saunas for several months.

On the day after surgery, your face and the incisions may be gently washed with soap and water. Scabs should be gently removed with a hydrogen peroxide-soaked Q-tip since their continued presence may prevent the formation of fine-line scars. Do not routinely clean incisions with hydrogen peroxide as this will cause irritation. Only use hydrogen peroxide to remove scabs. A very thin layer of Bacitracin antibiotic ointment should be applied with a Q-tip to all incisions on a daily basis. If irritation or a rash develops, discontinue the ointment and contact your doctor. Do not use Neosporin as it can redden the wound, thus mimicking an infection.

A feeling of numbness and tightness in your scalp, neck, cheeks and ears is common. This usually goes away within the first four to six weeks after surgery, but can last for six months to one year.

Your neck may feel very tight for six months or longer.

Forehead Lift or Brow Lift

Take it easy for the first two to three weeks after surgery.

Do not lift anything over 10 pounds, i.e. small children, groceries, and suitcases, for six weeks after surgery.

Avoid vigorous workouts for six weeks after surgery.

Do not play sports, i.e. tennis, golf, swimming, running, yoga, dance, or perform heavy house/yard work for six weeks after surgery.

Light cardio activity, i.e. walking moderate distances outside or light treadmill/stationary bike, may be resumed two weeks after surgery.

If you are employed, expect to take approximately seven to ten days off of work, as long as you remember that you may still have bruising that may be covered up with make-up for up to one month. It may take up to one month for your normal energy level to return.

Keep head elevated. Sleep with head on two pillows to reduce swelling.

Do not sleep on your stomach.

Swelling may affect cheeks and eyes for a week or so.

Ice compresses or a bag of frozen peas or corn may be applied to the forehead and eyes to help reduce swelling after your operation. Place a moist cloth or gauze over each eye, then place the cool pack on top of the cloth. Do not put ice directly on your eyelid skin. Leave the cool pack on the eyes for 20–30 minutes, and then remove it for 10 minutes. Repeat this as tolerated for the first 24 hours after surgery. Application of compresses after the first 24 hours does not usually further reduce swelling or discoloration.

As you heal, you may experience itching as your nerves regrow.

You may have some hair loss.

Do not use hair dye or permanent solution until approved by your surgeon.

Hair is generally shampooed on the second or third day after surgery. The area of sutures must be washed gently but thoroughly each time.

Do not set hair-dryer temperature on hot, as you may not have sensation in operated areas and thus you will not know if you are getting burned.

Makeup can be utilized to cover bruising three days after surgery. Do not apply makeup over the incisions. After the sutures are removed, you can use makeup on the incision areas.

When washing your face, be gentle—do not scrub.

For a classic lift, most stitches or clips are removed within fourteen days, sometimes in two stages. If bandages were used, they will be removed in one to two days.

For an endoscopic lift, stitches, or staples used to close the incisions are usually removed within a week.

Drains may be placed under the skin to remove excess fluid. They are connected to a plastic bulb, which generates suction. This is called a JP drain. If you are sent home with drains in place, secure them to the gauze necklace which the surgery recovery center may have provided—or use a shoelace or a bathrobe belt, knotted to make a necklace.

Bloody drainage into the bulb reservoir of the drain is normal. Excessive drainage, i.e. more than 50 cc/ml per eight-hour period, is abnormal. You should report this to your doctor promptly.

Hair Transplantation

It takes about five days for the grafts to take hold, and up to 18 months for full growth to occur.

Do not wash your hair for 24 to 48 hours after the procedure. The new follicles are very prone to damage in the early stages and washing could dislodge or damage them.

Scabs will form on your hair transplants post-op. This is a natural part of the healing process and these scabs should be left alone to heal on their own. Never pick or scrape the scabs as you risk infection or permanent damage to the new hair grafts.

Regular hair washing is important after the first two days after surgery. If you wash your hair as recommended, the chance of dislodging a graft is small. The shampooing helps remove dirt, blood, and oil, and will gently dislodge the crusts or scabs that form. These crusts should normally be gone within a few days to a week at the most. If they are not, you may not be shampooing effectively enough. Proper hygiene also helps prevent infection, and promotes the normal shedding of the transplanted hairs that occurs before they begin their new, relocated growth phase.

Keeping the recipient and donor areas moist promotes their healing. Saline solution or specific products, i.e. GraftCyte, sprayed on the grafts several times a day assists in the process. Any thick ointment, such as an antibiotic ointment, also works well for this.

While it may seem like your head spends an awful lot of time being wet in those first few days, it is actually very important not to let your hair soak in water for too long during your hair transplant post-op cleansing. New hair grafts that are immersed too long in water at one time may begin to swell as they soak up the excess water. This is evident when the grafts rise above the scalp and appear as little white bumps on the scalp.

For two weeks your hair transplant post-op regimen should include avoiding direct sun contact on your hair transplant as well as avoiding any strenuous exercise or contact sports.

It is good to keep the donor incision free of debris, crusts, and any accumulation of dirt and ointment. Vigorous rubbing or scratching is not allowed on the graft sites. This can easily dislodge grafts, which may cause mild bleeding, or lose one or more of those valuable hairs.

Sleep with your head elevated on at least two pillows.

Generally, the bulk of your hair transplant recovery time will be over after approximately one week.

Wearing a baseball cap will help protect the area if you are out in sun or public. Wear the cap loosely and do not fasten the strap on the back.

Lip Augmentation

Use ointment on your lips to keep them moist.

There may be a small dressing on the donor site—where the filler was obtained. It is common for the doctor to get the donor tissue from your pre-sacral area—the area right above your buttocks. Keep any donor-site dressings dry and intact on the evening after surgery. Notify your doctor if the dressing becomes loose or falls off. Cleaning the suture with a Q-tip dipped in hydrogen peroxide and then applying antibiotic ointment twice a day is an essential part of the healing process.

After 24 hours, keep incisions dry except for cleaning and ointment. Bathing or showering is okay as long as you don't get your incisions wet.

Sutures will be removed approximately five days after your surgery.

You should expect your lips to be very swollen and quite tender following your implant procedure.

Numbness may last for several days, and you may have difficulty drinking or eating without spilling a bit.

Advance diet from liquids to soft food, i.e. oatmeal, French toast, soup, and pasta, and then to your regular diet as tolerated.

Some doctors suggest avoiding dairy products for five days following lip augmentation surgery.

Sleep with the head of your bed elevated or use two or three pillows for one week after surgery.

No bending or straining and no lifting greater than 5 pounds, i.e. a gallon of milk.

Generally, makeup is not recommended until all incisions are healed. Hypoallergenic makeup is recommended. Always check with your doctor before applying any cosmetics, lotions, or sunscreens.

Always protect your face from the sun. A hat and sunglasses are recommended. Avoid prolonged, unprotected sun exposure for three months following lip augmentation procedures to prevent pigmentation of incision lines.

Nose Reshaping (Rhinoplasty)

Avoid strenuous activities or any activity that increases your blood pressure for two to three weeks after surgery.

Avoid body-contact sports, hitting or rubbing your nose, and sunglasses for two months after surgery.

Sleep with your head elevated on at least two pillows. Avoid sleeping on your stomach.

Contact lenses can be worn as soon as you feel like it, but glasses cannot be worn until your nose is completely healed—

approximately two months. After your nose splint is removed, tape your glasses to your forehead or prop them on your cheeks until completely healed.

A splint is applied immediately after surgery and is to be worn for seven days. Nasal packs—gauze packing placed inside your nostrils—may also be used. If you have nasal packing, it will be removed after a few days.

Temporary swelling and bruising around eyes and nose will increase at first and peak after two to three days. Most swelling and bruising should disappear within two weeks. Some subtle swelling—noticeable only to you—will remain for several months.

Some numbness may be present around the operative areas.

A small amount of bleeding is common during the first few days.

If nostrils are narrowed, sutures/stitches are removed in three to seven days. All other sutures either dissolve or are removed within two weeks.

The appearance of your nose improves in two to three weeks but the best results won't be seen for months to a year.

Your nasal tip drops to its permanent position in three to six months.

Massage to Decrease Swelling in the Face

The massage described on the next page should be performed after rhinoplasty, face lift, chin augmentation, lip augmentation, and forehead or brow lift. See Photo 1 to guide you when performing the massage techniques. This shows the directions in which you guide the fluid to the lymph nodes.

face massage

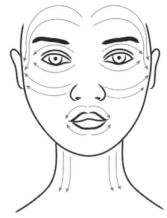

Photo 1: Direction of lymphatic massage of the face and neck
(courtesy of shutterstock.com)

Step 1. Pre-Treatment Massage

Perform in this order: collarbone, side of neck, back of neck, and deep breathing, all as described in Chapter 10 and below.

  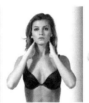 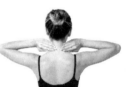

Photo 2A-D: Pre-treatment Massage

A. Deep breathing

Deep breathing is done by contracting the diaphragm.

Begin by placing both hands flat on your belly, over your diaphragm.

Inhale slowly—breathe deeply through your nose, allowing your stomach to expand.

As air enters your lungs, your abdomen—not your chest wall—should expand outwards.

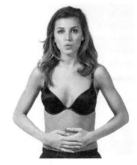

Photo 3: Deep breathing

Breathe out slowly through pursed lips, allowing your stomach to flatten.

Repeat five times with a short rest between each breath to avoid dizziness.

B. Collarbone (clavicle)

Place the bottom of your second (index) and third (middle) fingers on either side of your neck just above your collarbone.

Stroke down towards your collarbone and inward toward your neck. Stretch the skin just as far as it naturally goes. This stroke would look like two "J" strokes facing one another.

This technique can be applied on both sides at the same time or on one side at a time.

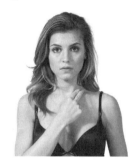

If doing both sides at the same time, you may find it more comfortable to cross your arms while you do this stroke.

Repeat 15 times.

Photo 4: Collarbone massage

C. Side of neck

Place the bottom of your hands on either side of your neck just under your ears and gently stretch the skin down towards your collarbone and release.

Keep a slow and rhythmic pace.

Repeat this stroke 10 to 15 times.

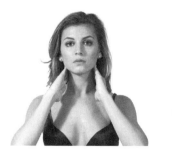 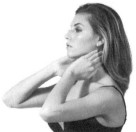

Photo 5A-B: Massaging the side of the neck

D. Back of neck

Place the bottom of your
hands on the back of your
neck just below your hairline
on either side of your spine.

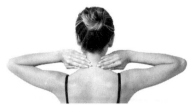

Photo 6: Massaging the back of the neck

Stretch the skin towards the
spine and then down toward base of neck and release.
Repeat 10 to 15 times.

Step 2. Around Ear

Place your pointer finger and thumb
gently on the soft tissue under your
jaw right below your ear. Place the
remainder of your three fingers in
front of your ear.

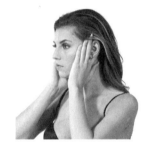

Twist your fingers toward your ear
five times.

Photo 7: Massaging the lymph
nodes around the ear

Give extra attention to the space behind your ear.

This technique is waking up the lymph nodes in the area
of the ear. This is where the swelling in the face will drain
towards and filter into the lymph nodes located around your ear.

Step 3. Under Jaw

Starting under your chin and stroking, under your jaw, down
towards your collarbone.

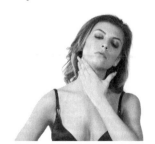
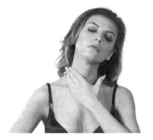

Photo 8A-B: Massage stroke under the jaw towards the collarbone.

Step 4. Chin

Place the pads of your fingers on the chin, below the lower lip and gently do circles that pull the skin down in the direction of your ear five times. Repeat this in two more positions: just to the side of the mouth and just above the upper lip.

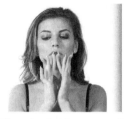 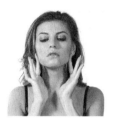

Photo 9A-B: Massage stroke from chin towards the ear.

Step 5. Upper Lip

Place the pads of your fingers below your upper lip. Gently make circles that pull your skin outwards, in the direction of your ear five times.

Repeat this in two different places, just to the side of your mouth and just above your upper lip.

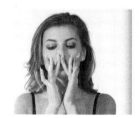 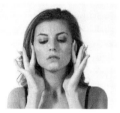

Photo 10A-B: Massage stroke from upper lip towards the ear

Step 6. Nose

Place the pads of your fingers just to the side of your nostrils. Gently make circles that pull your skin in the direction of your ear five times.

Repeat this in two different places, just to the side of the bridge of your nose and right below the inside edge of your eye.

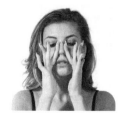

Photo 11: Massage stroke from nose towards the ear

Step 7. Cheeks

Start at the sides of your nose, just under your eyes, and massage out towards your ears.

Repeat this in order to massage the entire cheek.

Repeat this just below the cheekbones as well.

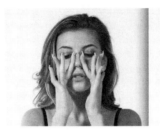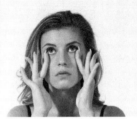

Photo 12A-B: Massage stroke from cheeks towards the ear

Step 8. Eyelids

Place all your fingertips just below your eye and stretch your skin gently toward your ears five times.

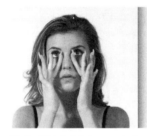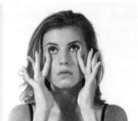

Photo 13A-B: Massage stroke from eyelids towards the ear

Step 9. Eyebrows

Gently pinching your eyebrows at the edge closest to your ears, pull towards your ears five times. Then gently stroke across the eyebrows, starting at the point closest to the bridge of your nose, and move outwards.

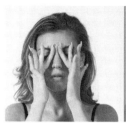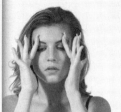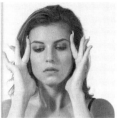

Photo 14A-C: Massage stroke from eyebrows towards the ear

Step 10. Forehead

Place the fingers of both hands on the center of your forehead and gently stretch down and outwards towards your ears five times.

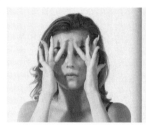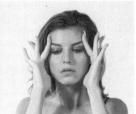

Photo 15A-B: Massage stroke from center of forehead towards the ear

Step 11. Top of Forehead

Gently place your hands at the top of your forehead at the hairline.

Putting pressure with the flats of your hands, gently pull from the center down towards your ears five times.

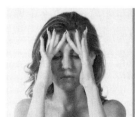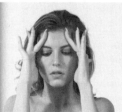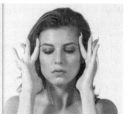

Photo 16A-C: Massage stroke from center of forehead, at the hairline, towards the ear

Chapter 15

Care of the Arms after Surgery

These are general recommendations—speak to your doctor about specific recommendations they may have regarding your procedure

Liposuction of the Arms

Do not lift anything greater than five pounds, i.e. a gallon of milk, for two weeks.

Activities involving the affected sites should be minimized for approximately two weeks.

Strenuous exercise and activities such as sports should be avoided for three to four weeks, depending on the extent of the surgery.

Do not play sports, i.e. tennis, golf, swimming, running, yoga, or dance, or perform heavy house/yard work for four weeks after surgery. Light cardio activity, i.e. walking moderate distances outside or treadmill/stationary bike, may be resumed two weeks after surgery.

You should sleep on your back during the immediate postoperative period. Prop your arms up with pillows so they are elevated at a level above your chest. This will help decrease the swelling and aid in your comfort level. Then progress to sleeping on your side. Normal sleeping positions are typically resumed two to three weeks after surgery.

Patients typically return to work after 10 days to two weeks.

You will be discharged wearing a pressure garment over the treated area. Most patients will wear pressure garment for six to eight weeks. The garment should be worn for 24 hours a day, including overnight, for six weeks after surgery. The garment may be washed on the gentle cycle as needed and air-dried. While this is being done, please stay off of your feet and minimize activity.

You will begin to get smaller as the swelling subsides. You may need to get a smaller compression garment. You can then switch to a sleeker compression garment after a few weeks.

Blood-tinged drainage staining your garment is normal.

If your incisions are oozing, place gauze on the area underneath your garment to provide compression.

You may shower the day after surgery. Wash all incisions gently with soap and water. If you have butterfly closures, i.e. Steri-Strips, on your incisions, leave them intact as they can get wet and normally will not come off in the shower. Remove your compression garment prior to showering and replace it when finished.

Please note that if you have a lot of swelling, it may be very difficult and painful to place your compression garment back on. If this is the case, you may want to wait two to three to shower.

After showering, re-apply pressure garment and gauze to protect areas of incisions.

Most of the swelling and discoloration usually subsides in six to eight weeks, but some may persist for six months or more.

Expect temporary numbness, bruising, swelling, soreness, burning sensation, bleeding, pain, and discomfort.

Bloody fluid draining from your incision sites is expected.

A drainage tube may be inserted beneath your skin during surgery to prevent fluid build-up.

You may feel stiff and sore for a few days.

Bruising may be apparent beyond the areas of liposuction, partially due to gravity.

The skin sutures/stitches are typically removed seven to 10 days after surgery. Suture removal is quick and uncomplicated. If you have butterfly closures on your incisions, these will remain in place for seven to 10 days.

Do not clean your incisions with hydrogen peroxide because it may kill wound-healing cells.

Do not apply hot or warm compresses to any of the surgical areas because it will increase swelling.

Fainting can occur at home after liposuction due to orthostatic hypotension resulting in syncope, which is fainting in response to a drop in blood pressure. You can prevent this by slowly removing post-op compression garments. Get assistance if you are having a difficult time. Take garments off one layer at a time, waiting a minute or two between removing the next garment. After urinating, stand up slowly. Have someone assist you when showering for the first time after liposuction. If feeling dizzy or lightheaded, immediately sit down and pump your ankles up and down. This will get your blood pressure back up. Be aware that there will blood-tinged drainage on your garments and leaking from incision sites. Don't be alarmed; this could cause you to faint. Do not remove the garments or shower on an empty stomach; this could cause hypoglycemia (low blood sugar). Hypoglycemia when performing these activities could cause you to faint.

Upper Arm Lift

Sleep on your back during the immediate postoperative period. Your arms will be wrapped with elastic bandages immediately after surgery to help minimize swelling. Prop both arms up with pillows so they are elevated at a level above your chest. This will help decrease swelling Normal sleeping positions can be resumed two to three weeks after surgery.

Some sutures/stitches will be absorbed. The remaining sutures will generally be removed in one to two weeks.

You will be required to purchase a compression garment before surgery—or it will be provided by your surgeon—that is specific for your procedure. The garment should be worn for 24 hours a day, including overnight, for four to six weeks after surgery. The garment may be washed on the gentle cycle and air-dried as needed. While this is being done, stay off your feet and minimize activity.

Your hands may swell. You can treat this with an elastic wrap or by wearing compression gloves. Elevating your arms and performing hand-pumping exercises will also combat hand swelling.

Do not play sports, i.e. tennis, golf, swimming, running, yoga, or dance, or perform heavy house/yard work for six weeks after surgery.

Do not lift anything over 10 pounds, i.e. small children, groceries, and suitcases, for six weeks after surgery.

Avoid vigorous workouts for six weeks after surgery.

Light cardio activity, i.e. walking moderate distances outside or light treadmill/stationary bike, may be resumed three weeks after surgery.

If you are employed, expect to take at least seven to 10 days off work.

Driving is permitted one to two weeks after surgery, when you have full range of motion and are able to drive without difficulty.

Massage to Decrease Swelling in the Arms

The massage described below should be performed after arm lift, liposuction of the arm, or any surgery that results in residual swelling of the upper extremities. See Photo 1 to guide you when performing the pre-treatment massage techniques. This shows the directions in which you guide the fluid to the lymph nodes.

Step 1. Pre-Treatment Massage

Perform in this order: collarbone, side of neck, back of neck, and deep breathing, all as described in Chapter 10 and below.

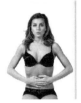 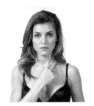 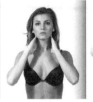 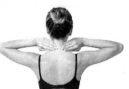

Photo 1A-D: Pre-treatment Massage

A. Deep breathing

Deep breathing is done by contracting the diaphragm.

Begin by placing both hands flat on your belly, over your diaphragm.

Inhale slowly—breathe deeply through your nose, allowing your stomach to expand into your hand.

As air enters your lungs, your abdomen—not your chest wall—should expand outwards.

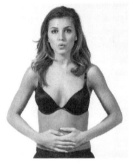

Breathe out slowly through pursed lips, allowing your stomach to flatten.

Repeat five times with a short rest between each breath to avoid dizziness.

Photo 2: Deep breathing

B. Collarbone (clavicle)

Place the bottom of your second (index) and third (middle) fingers on either side of your neck just above your collarbone.

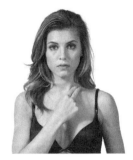

Stroke down towards your collarbone and inward toward your neck. Stretch the skin just as far as it naturally goes. This stroke would look like two "J" strokes facing one another.

Photo 4: Collarbone massage

This technique can be applied on both sides at the same time or on one side at a time.

If doing both sides at the same time, you may find it more comfortable
to cross your arms while you do this stroke.

Repeat 15 times.

C. Side of neck

Place the bottom of your hands on either side of your neck just under your ears and gently stretch the skin down towards your collarbone and release.

Keep a slow and rhythmic pace.

Repeat this stroke 10 to 15 times.

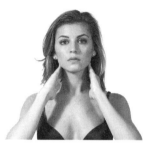

Photo 4: Massaging the side of the neck

D. Back of neck

Place the bottom of your hands on the back of your neck just below your hairline on either side of your spine.

Stretch the skin towards the spine and then down toward base of neck and release.

Repeat 10 to 15 times.

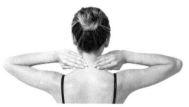

Photo 5: Massaging the back of the neck

Step 2. Stimulate Axillary Lymph Nodes

If the left arm is swollen, massage the left armpit/underarm.

If the right arm is swollen, massage the right armpit/underarm.

Perform in a circular motion. The pressure is directed downward, deep into the armpit and applied with the flats of fingers and palm.

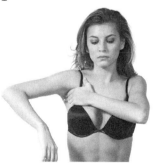

Photo 6: Massaging the armpit

Step 3. Upper Arm

Lymphatic fluid in the upper arm normally flows into the underarm. You want to direct the fluid to the axillary lymph nodes.

Starting with your shoulder, gently massage towards your neck. If it is not too much of a strain on your wrist, stroke across the back of your shoulder to your neck.

Try to gently stretch your skin towards your neck, then release.

Repeat 15 times.

Massage your whole upper arm from the inside of your arm to the top of your upper arm.

Repeat 15 times.

Now massage from the back of your arm to the top of your upper arm, stretching your skin, and then release.

Repeat 15 times.

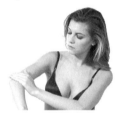 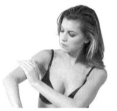 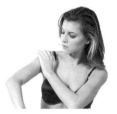

Photo 7A-C: Massaging the upper arm towards the shoulder elbow to the shoulder

Step 4. Forearm

Gently massage your wrist towards your elbow.

Then move to your upper arm towards the shoulder.

Gently stretching your skin, push fluid upwards and then release.

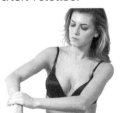 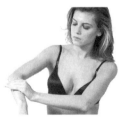 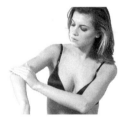

Photo 8A-C: Massaging forearm towards elbow

Step 5. Hand

Massage the back and palm of your hand.

Gently stretch the skin, towards the forearm, and then release.

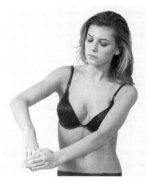

Photo 9: Massaging back and palm of hand towards forearm

Step 6. Fingers

Place your index finger and thumb of your unaffected hand on the base of your finger and gently stretch your skin towards your hand.

Massage the entire finger.

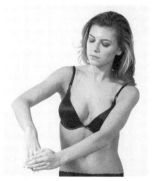

Photo 10: Massaging finger by stretching skin towards hand

Step 7. Go Back Up the Entire Arm

From the fingers, go to the top of the hand, wrist, forearm, upper arm, and finish at the shoulder.

Chapter 16

Care of the Breasts after Augmentation

These are general recommendations—speak to your doctor about specific recommendations they may have regarding your procedure

After Breast Augmentation

Wear a post-op garment, ACE wrap, or sports bra continuously, except while bathing, until you see your physician for your post-op appointment. After that, for at least three weeks after surgery you should wear a sports bra or a regular bra with no underwire.

Blood-tinged drainage staining your garment is normal.

You may shower 48 hours after surgery, but do not take any type of bath or dip in a tub, Jacuzzi, or pool.

Before showering, remove the ACE wrap and then carefully remove the pads. Leave the butterfly closures, i.e. Steri-Strips, in place. They can get wet—just pat them dry after you shower. Leave the butterfly closures on until you see your doctor for your post-op visit. If they fall off, clean the area with soap and water and pat dry.

Do not reapply the same pads. Always use fresh pads.

Do not lift your arms above 90 degrees—the level of your shoulder—for two weeks after surgery.

Do not lift more than five pounds, i.e. a gallon of milk, for about six weeks after surgery. This lifting restriction may prevent some women from returning to work.

It's a good idea to sleep with your head/trunk elevated to reduce swelling.

It's better not to sleep on your stomach.

You should begin walking immediately after surgery.

You should not perform any high-impact physical exercise for six to eight weeks after surgery. Such exercise, i.e. weight lifting, biking, jogging, and other forms of intense activities, may cause your implants to shift position or cause wound healing problems that may alter the appearance of your breasts after surgery.

You can resume low-impact exercise within two to three weeks.

You may start driving a car one week after surgery as long as you are no longer taking any pain medications.

Breast massage and postoperative exercises should be done daily as instructed by your doctor. These exercises typically begin after your first post-op doctor's appointment.

Capsular Contracture

What is Capsular Contracture?

Capsular contracture refers to a hardening of the breast pocket and scar tissue around a breast implant. When this happens, the breast implant is compressed, causing the breast to feel too hard and become misshapen. Symptoms of capsular contracture include hardness, swelling, and pain in your breast. Capsular contracture can be very painful and should be addressed as soon as possible.

Capsular contracture affects approximately five percent of women who have breast augmentation, but the specific rate of contracture is unknown.

Capsular contracture is the most frequent condition that leads to revision surgery after breast implant surgery. A capsular contracture typically develops three months after surgery, though it can develop at any time. Factors associated with capsular contracture formation include infection, hematoma, silicone bleed, and individual predisposition to hypertrophic scarring (big thick scar).

Here is a picture of a patient with capsular contracture after breast augmentation:

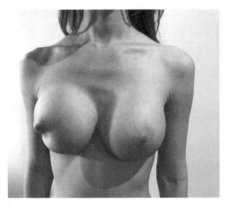

Photo 1: Example of Capsular contracture

Grading Capsular Contracture

For over 30 years, the Baker system has been a widespread, four-tier scale for grading capsule thickening or contracture.

Grade I. The breast has normal softness and appears natural in size and shape.

Grade II. The breast is a little firm but appears normal.

Grade III. The breast is firm and appears abnormal.

Grade IV. The breast is hard, painful to the touch, and appears abnormal.

Preventing Capsular Contracture

Prevention of capsular contraction is a joint effort between you and your surgeon. The technique your surgeon uses, the type of implant chosen, and placement of the implant are all factors that may affect the chances of developing a capsular contracture. Factors that you, as the patient, have greater control over include wearing your postoperative compression garment, following the specified exercise program, and performing postoperative massage.

The following measures may be included in your plan of care to prevent contractures:

External Methods

Topical medications

Vitamin E

MSM (methyl sulfonyl methane)

Papaverine

Accolate

Singulair

Mechanical techniques

Massage—see detailed discussion in the Massage to Prevent Capsular Contracture below

Clamps

Ultrasound

Diathermy

Internal Methods

Chemicals

Antibiotics

Steroids

Antiseptics

Structural

Textured surface

Polyurethane

Teflon (Gore Tex)

Alloderm

Silicone bleed barrier

Massage to Prevent Capsular Contracture

Regular breast massage in the first six months following surgery can reduce the risk for capsular contracture by moving your implants so that they can move freely within the implant pocket and retain the contour and symmetry of your breasts.

I teach my patients that implant massage helps to create a pocket that is larger than the implant itself. This helps the implant move around naturally inside its pocket and will create natural shape and motion, like a normal breast.

Breast massage also functions to some extent as a breast self-exam. Two studies found that women who developed potentially cancerous breast lumps found them earlier if they regularly massaged and felt their implants—proving that breast massage can be potentially life-saving.

When to Perform Breast Massage

Doctors typically recommend that you wait until after your one-week post-op visit to begin massage—get approval from your doctor before beginning any massage protocol.

Perform the following techniques as shown below, while lying down, at least twice each day for the first three months following surgery. While this may be uncomfortable when you first begin to perform the exercises, it is very important that you stick to them. After three months, if your breasts feel soft and the implants are moving freely, you may reduce your exercise and only perform your exercises one time a day.

After every day during the first year, you may perform your exercises once per day or every other day.

When Not to Perform Breast Massage

When your doctor advises against it. Every woman has a different medical history and therefore there may be certain circumstances that your doctor may feel you should not perform the breast massage. You should not perform breast massage if you begin to experience any of the following:

Any sharp pain in your breast

Hot or flushed skin over your breast

Severe tightening or hardness at any time with your breast implants

Severe pain to touch

Pus coming out from the incision or the nipple

Bloody drainage

Incision around the breast is separated and opening

Immediately stop the exercises and contact your doctor as soon as possible.

Massage Techniques

Technique 1

With your bra off, cup your breast directly under your nipple. The palm should push in and then roll up tightly against the chest wall. This causes the implant to rise upwards—watch for the implant to slide up as in the middle photograph.

To make sure the breasts are at the same level as when they were initially positioned, look in the mirror as you push both breasts.

Repeat this on each breast 10 times, holding for 10 seconds, three times a day.

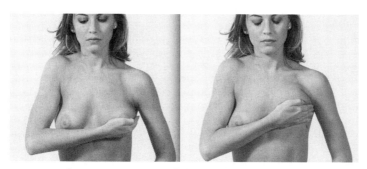

Photo 2A-B: Massage technique 1 after augmentation

Technique 2

This downward massage can be done less frequently as the implant settles over the weeks after surgery.

To make sure the breasts are at the same level as when they were initially positioned, look in the mirror as you push both breasts.

Repeat this on each breast 10 times, holding for 10 seconds, three times a day.

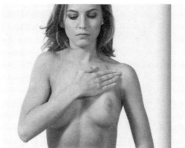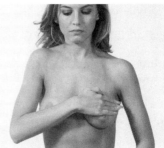

Photo 3A-B: Massage technique 2 after augmentation—downward push

Technique 3

This technique is used to address the sides of the implant.

Cup the outsides of your breast with your palms and simultaneously bring them together.

To make sure the breasts are evenly coming together, look in the mirror as you push both breasts.

Repeat this on each breast 10 times, holding for 10 seconds, three times a day.

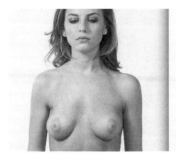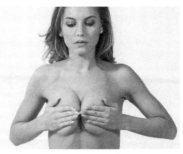

Photo 4A-B: Massage technique 3 after augmentation—
cupping sides and pushing breasts together

Technique 4

Circular massage technique, starting from the top and working in a clockwise pattern. Repeat in a counter clockwise pattern

Repeat this on each breast 10 times, three times a day.

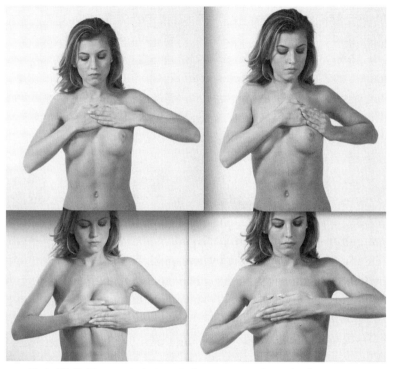

Photo 5A-D: Massage technique 4 after augmentation—circular massage

Kinesio Taping® for Treatment of Capsular Contracture

Let me begin by saying that this is an unconventional treatment I have designed for patients with capsular contracture, which has produced good results. Some doctors may find this unusual and may not agree with using this technique after breast augmentation surgery. The choice is yours.

What is Kinesio Taping®?

The Kinesio® taping method is designed to facilitate the body's natural healing process. It allows support and stability for muscles and joints without restricting their range of motion. It has been used to successfully treat a variety of orthopedic, neuromuscular, neurological, and medical conditions. Both Kinesio® Tex Tape and the training protocol have shown results that were unheard of using older methods and materials.

In the mid-1970s, Dr. Kenzo Kase, well-known licensed practitioner of chiropractic and acupuncture in the US and Japan, developed what has become Kinesio® tape in response to limitations he encountered in working with rigid sports-taping methods for his own patients. His product has a texture and elasticity very close to living human skin.

Dr. Kase had become familiar with a cryotherapy treatment for severe arthritis that utilized tape to adjust joint distortion. In Western medicine it had been assumed that once a joint is in a certain shape, it cannot be changed.

Dr. Kase was intrigued by the possibility that taping could improve joint distortion. He ordered supplies of the different athletic tapes that were then available. None of them gave him the results he was looking for. By trial and error, he realized that the source of the problem was actually in the muscle, not in the joint or in the bone. He saw that it was most effective to tape around the muscle to achieve joint correction. But the only tapes that he was able to obtain were rigid, designed to immobilize joints.

If injured or overused, a muscle loses its elasticity. Dr. Kase needed to develop a tape that would have the same elasticity as healthy human muscle. He knew from his practice that the tape would also need to stay on the skin after it was applied. He spent two years doing a lot of research on elasticity, adhesives, and breathability.

Finally, he invented what became Kinesio® Tex Tape—a tape that has the right amount of elasticity and also lifts the skin microscopically. Dr. Kase coined the name *Kinesio* to refer to body movement, as in kinesiology and kinesthesis.

Uses of Kinesio® Tex Tape

Neuromuscular re-education

Pain reduction

Performance optimization

Injury prevention

Improving circulation and healing

Kinesio® tape comes in rolls, from which strips can be cut to desired lengths. It also comes in pre-cut strips for ease of use.

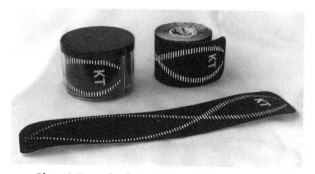

Photo 6: Example of Kinesio® tape in the color black

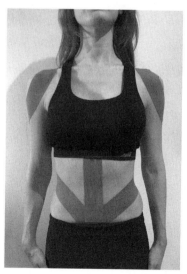

Photo 7: Example of applications of Kinesio® tape

Kinesio® Taping and Capsular Contracture

After breast augmentation surgery, capsular contractures can sometimes occur. Kinesio® taping can be used in combination with massage, proper medication, and topical creams to treat the contracture as best as possible. What typically happens when the contracture occurs in one breast is that the breast moves upward and/or outward. The tape can be worn for several days at a time to hold the breasts in place.

Here is a picture of that patient with the tape holding the breasts in a good position:

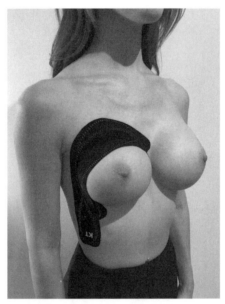

Photo 8: Example of applications of Kinesio® tape application after breast augmentation

Chapter 17

Care of the Chest and Torso after Surgery

These are general recommendations—speak to your doctor about specific recommendations they may have regarding your procedure

Abdominoplasty (Tummy Tuck)

Your doctor may advise you to bend your legs at your hips while resting and relaxing in bed to reduce strain on the abdominal wall muscles for the first two days after surgery.

Maintain a slightly flexed posture when walking, for approximately one week. Then begin to gradually straighten to an upright posture.

Sleep with your head slightly elevated and with pillows under your knees to decrease the tension on your incision.

No lifting or straining, but if you must pick something up, bend your knees, keeping your trunk and head upright.

After surgery, you will wear an abdominal binder for the first two weeks. After two weeks, you can then switch to a sleeker garment, i.e. Spanx®.

Wear a compression garment for at least four to six weeks.

Blood-tinged drainage staining your garment is normal.

If your incision is oozing, place gauze on the area underneath your garment to provide extra compression.

The JP (Jackson-Pratt) drain helps remove excess blood and fluid from under the skin at the incision site. The drain will stay in place for approximately one week or until the drainage has slowed down or stopped.

After healing occurs, the draining fluid will change color—it starts out red and gradually turns yellow.

Keep the drain pinned to your clothing/binder to keep the drain from being pulled out.

Empty the drain at least twice a day and keep track of how much fluid you dump out each time.

Gently clean around each drain with mild soap and water, rinse well, and keep the area dry.

Abdominal drains will be removed when your doctor decides it is time to do so.

Keep incisions clean and inspect them daily for signs of infection.

Place sterile, non-stick dressings over incisions and around drain sites to absorb moisture and to prevent irritation by your garment along the incision line.

Surface stitches/sutures may be dissolvable. If they are not dissolvable, they are typically removed in seven to 10 days.

Take a sponge bath daily until drains are removed.

You may shower 48 hours after removal of all drainage tubes.

No tub soaking while sutures or drains are in place

No lifting or straining for two weeks following surgery.

No heavy lifting for approximately six weeks. This means not lifting anything more than five pounds, i.e. a gallon of milk.

Get plenty of rest for the first seven to 10 days after surgery.

Exercises that work the abdominal muscles should be avoided for at least three months.

Low-impact exercise can be resumed within two to three weeks. High-impact exercise should be avoided for at least six to eight weeks.

Resume sexual activity as comfort permits, usually two to three weeks after surgery.

Do not return to work until the drains are removed, usually about 10 days after surgery.

Typically, patients return to work in two to four weeks.

Do not drive until you have full range of arm motion and are no longer taking pain medication.

Breast Lift

Crescent lifts and donut lifts will heal far more quickly and with less discomfort than techniques which make more than one incision in the breast.

Sensitivity in the breasts or nipples might be temporarily reduced or lost. Most of this sensation should come back slowly over the next few days or weeks. Some permanent loss of sensation is possible, although complete permanent loss of feeling is rare.

Generally, immediately after surgery, you can expect to be bandaged, wearing compression garments, plus you may have some surgical drains.

Wear your surgical bra 24/7 for six weeks after surgery unless your doctor tells you otherwise.

Leave your dressing on for length of time prescribed by your doctor.

If drainage tubes have been placed, you may shower for the first time 48 hours after they are removed.

Keep incisions clean and inspect them daily for signs of infection.

Generally, stitches will be removed in stages over a period of approximately three weeks, beginning about one week after surgery.

Limit the use of your arms for four to six weeks.

Do not lift your arms above 90 degrees—shoulder height—for two weeks.

No heavy lifting for approximately six weeks. This includes anything greater than five pounds, i.e. a gallon of milk.

Avoid strenuous exercise and activities for four to six weeks.

Do not drive a car for two weeks. After two weeks, only drive a car with an automatic shift and power steering. Do not drive if you are still taking pain medication. Do not drive until you have full range of motion with your arms.

Social and work activities can be resumed in one to two weeks, depending on your type of work).

You may want to sleep with your head/trunk elevated to reduce swelling.

It's best not to sleep on your stomach.

Breast Reduction

Immediately after surgery, you may not have sensation in the nipples. This usually returns as your body recovers.

Your first menstruation following surgery may cause your breasts to swell and hurt.

You may have random, shooting pains for a few months.

You will be discharged from surgery with a drainage tube in each breast. Generally, drainage tubes will be removed when the drainage is less than 30 ccs/mls over a period of one to two days—your doctor decides.

Wear your surgical bra 24/7 or as directed for six weeks after surgery.

Your surgeon may let you move into a sports bra 24/7 after two weeks. The bra needs to be a front closure with formed cups, not a flat front.

Avoid bras with stays and underwires for four to six weeks.

You may shower 48 hours after removal of the drainage tubes.

Keep incisions clean and inspect them daily for signs of infection.

You may pad the incisions with gauze for comfort.

If your breast skin is exceedingly dry after surgery, you can apply a moisturizer several times a day, but be sure to keep the stitches/suture area dry.

Avoid lifting anything over five pounds, i.e. more than a gallon of milk, for two weeks.

Refrain from vigorous activity for two to six weeks. Increase activity gradually as tolerated.

Do not drive until you have full range of motion with your arms or if you are still taking pain medication.

Most people resume work in about two weeks, if their work is not too strenuous.

You may want to sleep with your head/trunk elevated to reduce swelling.

It's best not to sleep on your stomach.

Liposuction of the Chest, Abdomen, Flanks, or Back

At the time of surgery, you will be placed in a well-fitting compression garment, which should be worn for 24 hours a day (including overnight) for at least six weeks after surgery. Your garment will have vents so that it may be worn even when using the toilet. The garment may be washed on the gentle cycle and air-dried as needed. While this is being done, please stay off of your feet and minimize activity.

Your will begin to get smaller as the swelling subsides. You may need to get a smaller compression garment. You can then switch to a sleeker compression garment, i.e. Spanx®, after a few weeks.

Blood-tinged drainage staining your garment is normal.

If your incision is oozing, place gauze on the area underneath your garment to provide extra compression.

You may shower the day after surgery. Wash all incisions gently with soap and water. If you have butterfly closures, i.e. Steri-Strips, on your incisions, leave them intact as they can get wet and normally will not come off in the shower. Remove your compression garment prior to showering, and replace it when finished.

Re-apply pressure garment and gauze to cover areas of incisions. Please note that if you have a lot of swelling, it may be very difficult and painful to place your compression garment back on. If this is the case, you may want to wait two or three days to shower.

Most of the swelling and discoloration usually subsides in six to eight weeks, but some may persist for six months or more.

Expect temporary numbness, bruising, swelling, soreness, burning sensation, bleeding, pain, and discomfort.

A drainage tube may be inserted beneath the skin during surgery to prevent fluid build-up.

You will have small incision sites at the point of introduction of the instrument used to remove the fat tissue.

After surgery, you may feel stiff and sore for a few days.

Bruising may be apparent beyond the areas of liposuction, partially due to gravity.

Skin sutures/stitches are typically removed seven to 10 days after surgery. Suture removal is quick and uncomplicated. If you have butterfly closures on your incisions, these will remain in place for seven to 10 days.

Do not clean your incisions with hydrogen peroxide because it may kill wound-healing cells.

Do not apply hot or warm compresses to any of the surgical areas because they will increase swelling.

Fainting (vasovagal syncope) can occur at home after liposuction due to a drop in blood pressure. Here are ways you can prevent this:

Slowly remove compression garments. Get assistance if you
are having a difficult time.

Take garments off one layer at a time, waiting a minute or
two between removing the next garment.

Stand up slowly after urinating.

Have someone assist you when showering for the first time
after liposuction.

If you feel dizzy or lightheaded, immediately sit down and
pump your ankles up and down. This will raise your blood
pressure back up.

Be aware that there will blood-tinged drainage on your
garments and leaking from incision sites. Becoming alarmed
about this could cause you to faint.

Do not remove the garments or shower on an empty stomach
as this could cause hypoglycemia. Hypoglycemia when
performing these activities could cause you to faint.

Do not lift anything heavier than five pounds, i.e. a gallon
of milk, for the first two weeks after surgery.

Activities involving the affected sites should be minimized
for approximately two weeks.

Strenuous exercise and activities such as sports should be
avoided for three to four weeks, depending on the extent of
the surgery.

Do not play sports, i.e. tennis, golf, swimming, or running,
do yoga or dance, or perform heavy house/yard work for four
weeks after surgery.

Light cardio activity, i.e. walking moderate distances outside
or light treadmill/stationary bike, may be resumed two weeks
after surgery.

You should sleep on your back after surgery. If your arms
and/or legs were operated on, prop them up with pillows so
they are elevated at a level above your chest. This will help
decrease swelling. If your trunk was operated on, prop your
back up with pillows so you bend slightly at the waist. This

will aid in your comfort level. Then progress to sleeping on your side. Normal sleeping positions are typically resumed two to three weeks after surgery.

Patients typically return to work after 10 days to two weeks.

Lower Body Lift

After surgery you will have multiple drains in place to prevent an accumulation of blood (hematoma) or fluid (seroma). Most drains will be removed between the third and seventh days, though some will remain in place for up to two weeks.

Do not stand fully upright: If your body lift included your abdomen, you must not stand fully upright. Standing upright could greatly affect your results and could cause serious injury. A walker or cane may be used for assistance.

Rest, but not bed rest. While rest is important in the early stages of healing, equally important is that you are keep moving, meaning that you walk under your own strength. As you recover, spend ten minutes every two hours engaged in light walking indoors.

It is important to rest for six weeks after surgery. While it is rare to tear the skin stitches, it is possible to loosen the underlying permanent abdominal, thigh, and buttock stitches, which will decrease the positive effects of the surgery. It is important to avoid all heavy lifting or exercise during the first six weeks after surgery while all levels of your tissues are healing and forming new collagen scar fibers.

A recliner chair may make it easier for you to get up and down from a lying position.

Your incisions will seep fluid and some blood for a short time after surgery. Carefully follow the instructions for drain care and record drained fluid on the drain care log which will be provided to you prior to discharge after surgery.

Two to seven days after surgery, as directed by your doctor, take a warm but not hot shower. Do not take a bath. Limit your shower to 10 minutes and use antibacterial soap, i.e. Lever 2000 or Dial. Do not rub your incisions. You should cleanse around the drain sites two to three times a day with cotton swabs, moistened with hydrogen peroxide. Apply Bacitracin ointment over the incisions with a clean Q-tip, and then wrap the incisions lightly with 4" x 4" gauze. Apply a fragrance-free moisturizer to the surrounding skin—but not on your incisions or sutures/stitches. Your compression garment will hold all of the dressings in place.

Wear your compression garment or elastic wraps 24/7, removing them only to cleanse your incision or to empty drains. Wear your garment for about four to six weeks.

Pectoral Implants

Unlike female breast implant surgery, pectoral implants do not carry the risk of breaking and/or leaking. The silicone implants used for men is soft but solid, i.e. not filled with liquid.

During the recovery period, you should not lift your arms. This allows the implants to settle into the fascia pockets that surround the muscle.

Due to the stress placed on the pectoral muscles during usual everyday activities, i.e. lifting or arm extension, pectoral implants are usually subjected to intense movement. Thus, the possibility of an implant shifting or moving after surgery is a concern.

When the dressings are removed, follow the prescribed gentle exercise program for the next few weeks to permit a full and comfortable range of motion of your arms. This allows the implants to settle into the fascia pockets that surround the muscle.

Generally, within a week or two, physical use of the upper body muscles may be resumed. Usually within one month, exercise level may be advanced to full pectoral muscular activity.

Direction for Massage Strokes

See the image below to guide you when performing the massage techniques for the abdomen, chest and back. This shows the directions in which you guide the fluid to the lymph nodes.

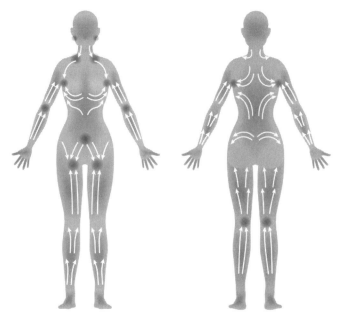

Photo 1: Direction of massage for the chest, abdomen and back
(courtesy of shutterstock.com)

Massage Treatment to Decrease Swelling in the Abdomen

The next steps treat the lymphatic vessels of the deep abdomen, located beneath the abdominal muscles. These treatments are for the following: liposuction of the abdomen, abdominoplasty, body lift, breast implants, or any abdominal surgery.

Step 1. Pre-Treatment Massage

Perform in this order: collarbone, side of neck, back of neck, and deep breathing.

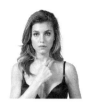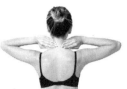

Photo 2A-D: Pre-treatment Massage

A. Deep breathing

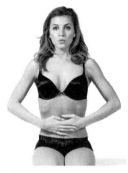

Deep breathing is done by contracting the diaphragm.

Begin by placing both hands flat on your belly, over your diaphragm.

Inhale slowly—breathe deeply through your nose, allowing your stomach to expand into your hand.

Photo 3: Deep breathing

As air enters your lungs, your abdomen—not your chest wall—should expand outwards.

Breathe out slowly through pursed lips, allowing your stomach to flatten.

Repeat five times with a short rest between each breath to avoid dizziness.

B. Collarbone (clavicle)

Place the bottom of your second (index) and third (middle) fingers on either side of your neck just above your collarbone.

Stroke down towards your collarbone and inward toward your neck. Stretch the skin just as far as it naturally goes. This stroke would look like two "J" strokes facing one another.

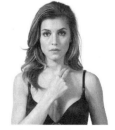

This technique can be applied on both sides at the same time or on one side at a time.

If doing both sides at the same time, you may find it more comfortable to cross your arms while you do this stroke.

Photo 4: Collarbone massage

Repeat 15 times.

C. Side of neck

Place the bottom of your hands on either side of your neck just under your ears and gently stretch the skin down towards your collarbone and release.

Keep a slow and rhythmic pace.

Repeat this stroke 10 to 15 times.

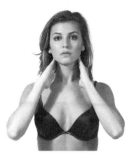

Photo 5: Massaging the side of the neck

D. Back of neck

Place the bottom of your hands on the back of your neck just below your hairline on either side of your spine.

Stretch the skin towards the spine and then down toward base of neck and release.

Repeat 10 to 15 times.

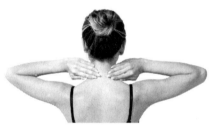

Photo 6: Massaging the back of the neck

Step 2. Massage Armpit Lymph Nodes

To prepare to redirect fluid from the abdomen, you begin by placing your palm inside each armpit.

Knead your palm firmly in a counterclockwise circle.

Pressure is applied with the flat surfaces of your fingers and palm, and is directed downward, deep into the armpit.

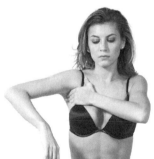

Photo 7: Stimulating the axillary nodes

Perform this in each armpit about 10 to 15 times.

Step 3. Massage Upper Abdomen

Place your flat fingers on the middle of your stomach, in the middle of your stomach, right above your belly button.

Push your hand gently towards the outside of your torso, stretching your skin, as far as it naturally goes, away from the middle of your body.

Repeat this motion 10 to 15 times, slowly moving your hand placement closer towards the outside of your body.

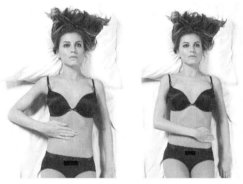

Photo 8A-B: Massage the upper abdomen above the belly button

Next start on the outside of your torso and drag your hand up the side of your body towards your armpit, stretching your skin, as far as it naturally goes, and then release.

Use the opposite hand of it is easier.

Repeat this motion 10 to 15 times, slowly moving your hand placement closer towards the armpit.

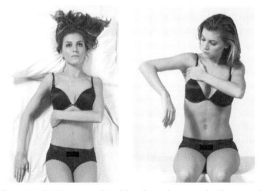

Photo 9A-B: Massage the side of trunk towards the armpit

Step 4. Massage Groin and Outer Thigh Lymph Nodes

Place your hand on the angle that forms between your leg and pelvis (the underwear line).

Place your fingertips on this crease.

Your hand is placed just below the hipbone, but closer to your private area.

Make circles for two to three minutes, directing the pressure toward your belly.

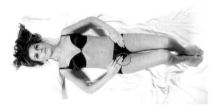
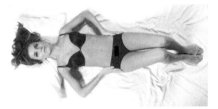

Photo 10A: Massaging the groin lymph nodes

Photo 10B: Massaging the outer thigh lymph nodes

Step 5. Massage Lower Abdomen

Place your flat fingers on the middle of your stomach, in the middle of your stomach, right below your belly button.

Push your hand gently towards the outside of your hips, stretching your skin, as far as it naturally goes, away from the middle of your body.

Repeat this motion 10 to 15 times, slowly moving your hand placement closer towards the outside of your body.

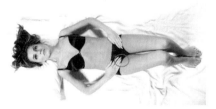
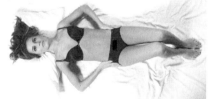

Photo 11A-B: Massage the lower abdomen below the belly button

Step 6. Massage Pubic Area

Next start in the middle of your pubic area, stretching your skin, as far as it naturally goes, and then release.

Move your hands out towards the groin lymph nodes.

Repeat this motion 10 to 15 times, slowly moving your hand placement closer towards the hip bones.

Massage Treatment to Decrease Swelling in the Chest

This should be performed after breast implants, pectoral implants, liposuction of the abdomen/flanks, body lift, or any upper body surgery. This technique can also be done before treatment of the arms for additional benefits.

Step 1. Perform Pre-Treatment Massage

Perform in this order: collarbone, side of neck, back of neck, and deep breathing.

   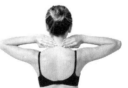

Photo 12A-D: Pre-treatment Massage

A. Deep breathing

Deep breathing is done by contracting the diaphragm.

Begin by placing both hands flat on your belly, over your diaphragm.

Inhale slowly—breathe deeply through your nose, allowing your stomach to expand into your hand.

As air enters your lungs, your abdomen—not your chest wall—should expand outwards.

Breathe out slowly through pursed lips, allowing your stomach to flatten.

Repeat five times with a short rest between each breath to avoid dizziness.

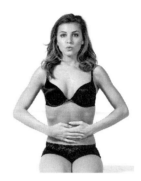

Photo 13: Deep breathing

B. Collarbone (clavicle)

Place the bottom of your second (index) and third (middle) fingers on either side of your neck just above your collarbone.

Stroke down towards your collarbone and inward toward your neck. Stretch the skin just as far as it naturally goes. This stroke would look like two "J" strokes facing one another.

This technique can be applied on both sides at the same time or on one side at a time.

If doing both sides at the same time, you may find it more comfortable to cross your arms while you do this stroke.

Repeat 15 times.

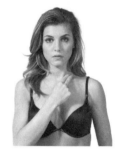

Photo 14: Collarbone massage

C. Side of neck

Place the bottom of your hands on either side of your neck just under your ears and gently stretch the skin down towards your collarbone and release.

Keep a slow and rhythmic pace.

Repeat this stroke 10 to 15 times.

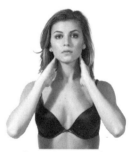

Photo 15: Massaging the side of the neck

D. Back of neck

Place the bottom of your hands on the back of your neck just below your hairline on either side of your spine.

Stretch the skin towards the spine and then down toward base of neck and release.

Repeat 10 to 15 times.

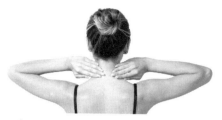

Photo 16: Massaging the back of the neck

Step 2. Massage the Armpit Lymph Nodes

To prepare to redirect fluid from the chest, you begin by placing your palm inside each armpit.

Knead your palm firmly in a counterclockwise circle.

Pressure is applied with the flat surfaces of your fingers and palm, and is directed downward, deep into the armpit.

Perform this in each armpit about 10 to 15 times.

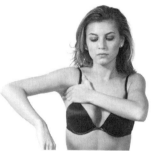

Photo 17: Massaging the armpit/underarm

Step 3. Treatment of the Chest

Place your fingers on your breast bone (sternum), in the middle of your chest above one breast.

Push your hand gently towards your opposite armpit, stretching your skin, as far as it naturally goes, and then release.

Repeat this motion 10 to 15 times, slowly moving your hand placement closer towards the armpit.

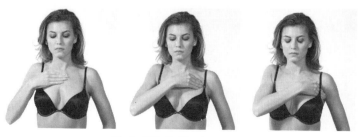

Photo 18A-C: Chest massage

Massage Treatment to Decrease Swelling in the Back

The next steps treat the lymphatic vessels of the deep abdomen, located beneath the abdominal muscles. These treatments are for the following: liposuction of the back, body lift, or any cosmetic procedure of the back.

Step 1. Pre-Treatment Massage

Perform in this order: collarbone, side of neck, back of neck, and deep breathing.

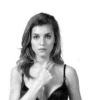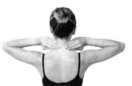

Photo 19A-D: Pre-treatment Massage

A. Deep breathing

Deep breathing is done by contracting the diaphragm.

Begin by placing both hands flat on your belly, over your diaphragm.

Inhale slowly—breathe deeply through your nose, allowing your stomach to expand into your hand.

As air enters your lungs, your abdomen—not your chest wall—should expand outwards.

Breathe out slowly through pursed lips, allowing your stomach to flatten.

Repeat five times with a short rest between each breath to avoid dizziness.

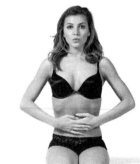

Photo 20: Deep breathing

B. Collarbone (clavicle)

Place the bottom of your second (index) and third (middle) fingers on either side of your neck just above your collarbone.

Stroke down towards your collarbone and inward toward your neck. Stretch the skin just as far as it naturally goes. This stroke would look like two "J" strokes facing one another.

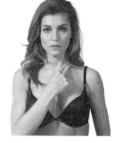

This technique can be applied on both sides at the same time or on one side at a time.

If doing both sides at the same time, you may find it more comfortable to cross your arms while you do this stroke.

Repeat 15 times.

Photo 21: Collarbone massage

C. Side of neck

Place the bottom of your hands on either side of your neck just under your ears and gently stretch the skin down towards your collarbone and release.

Keep a slow and rhythmic pace.

Repeat this stroke 10 to 15 times.

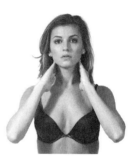

Photo 22: Massaging the side of the neck

D. Back of neck

Place the bottom of your hands on the back of your neck just below your hairline on either side of your spine.

Stretch the skin towards the spine and then down toward base of neck and release.

Repeat 10 to 15 times.

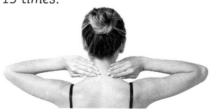

Photo 23: Massaging the back of the neck

Step 2. Massage Groin and Outer Thigh Lymph Nodes

Place your hand on the angle that forms between your leg and pelvis (the underwear line).

Place your fingertips on this crease.

Your hand is placed just below the hipbone, but closer to your private area.

Make circles for two to three minutes, directing the pressure toward your belly.

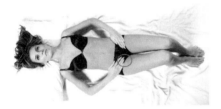

Photo 24A: Massaging the groin lymph nodes

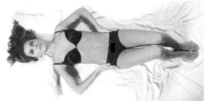

Photo 24B: Massaging the outer thigh lymph nodes

Step 3. Massage Lower Back

*For this section it may be easier to have someone perform on you

Place your flat fingers on the middle of your lower back, along your spine.

Pull your hands gently out towards the sides of your torso, stretching your skin, as far as it naturally goes, away from the middle of your body.

Repeat this motion 10 to 15 times, slowly moving your hand placement closer towards the outside of your body.

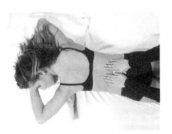
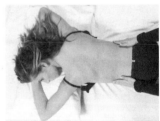

Photo 25A-B: Massage the lower back

Step 4. Massage Armpit Lymph Nodes

To prepare to redirect fluid from the back, you begin by placing your palm inside each armpit.

Knead your palm firmly in a counterclockwise circle.

Pressure is applied with the flat surfaces of your fingers and palm, and is directed downward, deep into the armpit.

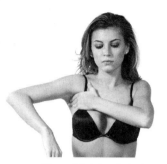

Photo 26: Stimulating the axillary nodes

Perform this in each armpit about 10 to 15 times.

Step 5. Massage Upper Back

For this section it may be easier to have someone perform on you

Place your flat fingers on the middle of your back, along the spine.

Pull your hands gently out towards the sides of your torso, stretching your skin, as far as it naturally goes, away from the middle of your body.

Repeat this motion 10 to 15 times, slowly moving your hand placement closer towards the outside of your body.

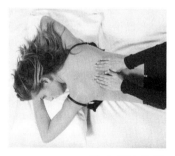 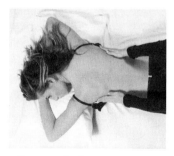

Photo 27A-B: Massage the upper back

Next start on the outside of your torso and drag your hand up the side of your body towards your armpit, stretching your skin, as far as it naturally goes, and then release.

Use the opposite hand of it is easier.

Repeat this motion 10 to 15 times, slowly moving your hand placement closer towards the armpit.

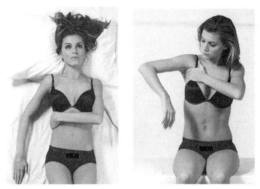

Photo 28A-B: Massage the side of trunk towards the armpit

Chapter 18

Care of the Buttocks and Legs after Surgery

These are general recommendations—speak to your doctor about specific recommendations they may have regarding your procedure

Buttock Implants

Postoperative days 1 through 7: You may not sit or lay on your buttocks or the grafted area, except for sitting to use the toilet.

Days 8 through 14: You may sit up for to five minutes twice a day.

Days 15 through 21: You may sit up for to nine minutes, five times a day.

Day 22 and after: You may sit as long as you are comfortable.

It is recommended that you sleep on your stomach or your side.

You should wear your garment 24/7 for at least four weeks after surgery.

Walk frequently, starting the first day after surgery.

While in bed, point and flex your feet at the ankles—ankle pumping—to prevent blood clots from forming.

Proper hygiene is essential. After a bowel movement or after voiding, take great care not to wipe towards the wound.

Most patients typically require two weeks off work after surgery.

Do not return to any exercise other than walking for at least six weeks.

Buttock Lift

Your garment should be worn for approximately six weeks.

Do not shower until 48 hours after the drainage tubes are removed.

Do not sit for one week after surgery.

Most people can return to work two to three weeks after surgery, provided their work does not involve extensive sitting.

It is recommended that you sleep on your stomach or your side.

Avoid strenuous exercise and activities, i.e. sports, for at least for at least four to six weeks.

There may be numbness around the operative areas.

You may shower two days after your surgery.

Gently wash the incision area and pat it dry, being careful not to rub the incisions.

Do not take a bath for two weeks after surgery.

Do not soak in a hot tub or swim for two weeks after surgery—longer if you have any signs of an infection.

Calf Augmentation

Most people return to work in seven to 10 days.

Avoid strenuous activities for four to six weeks after surgery. Usually after six weeks, you can return to full-play sports and other normal physical activities.

During the first two days after surgery, someone should assist you when you get up to go to the bathroom and your legs should be elevated as often as possible to reduce swelling and discomfort.

Your dressings can be removed on the second day after surgery.

Starting on the second day after surgery, you should begin walking around the house. You may also start taking brief showers.

You can expect to walk stiffly for the first week or so, but you are encouraged to gradually walk greater distances.

Normal walking starts to return during the second and third week after surgery.

Your skin will start to stretch and its bruised and shiny appearance will start to fade.

Activities such as running, biking, and weight-lifting should be avoided until one or two months after surgery, depending on your comfort level.

Full return to normal activities usually occurs after four to six weeks.

Liposuction of the Thighs

Do not lift anything greater than five pounds, i.e. a gallon of milk, for two weeks.

Activities involving the affected sites should be minimized for approximately two weeks.

Strenuous exercise and activities such as sports should be avoided for three to four weeks, depending on the extent of the surgery.

Do not play sports, i.e. tennis, golf, swimming, running, yoga, or dance, or perform heavy house/yard work for four weeks after surgery.

Light cardio activity, i.e. walking moderate distances outside or treadmill/stationary bike, may be resumed two weeks after surgery.

You should sleep on your back immediately after surgery. Prop your legs up with pillows so they are elevated at a level above your chest. This will help decrease swelling and aid in your comfort level.

Then progress to sleeping on your side. Normal sleeping positions are typically resumed two to three weeks after surgery.

Patients typically return to work after seven days to two weeks.

At the time of surgery, you will be placed in a well-fitting compression garment, which should be worn for 24 hours a day, including overnight, for six weeks after surgery. Your garment will have vents so that it may be worn even when using the restroom.

The garment may be washed on the gentle cycle and air-dried as needed. While this is being done, stay off of your feet and minimize activity.

You will begin to get smaller as the swelling subsides. You may need to get a smaller compression garment. You can then switch to a sleeker compression garment, i.e. Spanx®, after a few weeks.

Blood-tinged drainage staining your garment is normal.

If your incision is oozing, place gauze on the area underneath your garment to provide extra compression.

You may shower the day after surgery. Wash all incisions gently with soap and water. If you have butterfly closures, i.e. Steri-Strips, on your incisions, leave them intact. They can get wet and normally will not come off in the shower. Remove your compression garment prior to showering and replace it when finished.

Please note that if you have a lot of swelling, it may be very difficult and painful to place your compression garment back on. If this is the case, you may want to wait two or three days to shower.

After showering, cover the incision areas with gauze to protect them, and then replace your pressure garment.

Most of the swelling and discoloration usually subsides in six to eight weeks, but some may persist for six months or more.

Expect temporary numbness, bruising, swelling, soreness, burning sensation, bleeding, pain, and discomfort.

Drainage of bloody fluid from incision sites is expected.

A drainage tube may be inserted beneath the skin during surgery to prevent fluid build-up.

You may feel stiff and sore for a few days.

Bruising may be apparent beyond the areas of liposuction, partially due to gravity.

The skin sutures/stitches are typically removed seven to 10 days after surgery. Suture removal is quick and uncomplicated. Butterfly closures, i.e. Steri-Strips, will remain intact for seven to 10 days.

Do not clean your incisions with hydrogen peroxide because it may kill wound-healing cells.

Do not apply hot or warm compresses to any of the surgical areas because they will increase swelling.

Fainting—due to orthostatic hypotension—can occur at home after liposuction due to a drop in blood pressure. You can prevent this by slowly remove post-op compression garments. Get assistance if you are having a difficult time. Take garments off one layer at a time, waiting a minute or two between removing the next garments. After urinating, stand up slowly to prevent fainting. Having someone assist you when showering for the first time after liposuction will also keep you from feeling faint.

If feeling dizzy or lightheaded, immediately sit down and pump your ankles up and down. This will get your blood pressure back up.

Be aware that there will be blood-tinged drainage on your garments and leaking from incision sites. Don't be alarmed by this. Being alarmed could cause you to faint.

Do not remove the garments or shower on an empty stomach as this could cause hypoglycemia (low blood sugar). Hypoglycemia when performing these activities could cause you to faint.

Thigh Lift

Full extension—standing up fully—may not be possible during the first week after surgery.

It is actually better if you stand and walk than just sit for two weeks.

Sleep on your stomach for the first two weeks after surgery. Put two or three pillows under your tummy and knees or lower legs to make it more comfortable for you to sleep on your stomach.

You should also sleep with your feet elevated to minimize swelling. Normal sleeping positions can be resumed two to three weeks after surgery.

Try to avoid excessive straining when you have a bowel movement.

It is not uncommon for your genitals, legs, and feet to become swollen and/or bruised after surgery. If this becomes excessive, contact your doctor.

Do not attempt to do any work around the house. Avoid bending over, lifting, or straining.

Avoid lifting or carrying any more than five pounds, i.e. a gallon of milk, for six weeks.

Do not play sports, i.e. tennis, golf, swimming, or running, or do yoga or dance, or perform heavy house work or yard work for six weeks after surgery.

Light cardio activity, i.e. walking moderate distances outside or light treadmill/stationary bike, may be resumed three weeks after surgery.

At the time of surgery, you will be placed in a well-fitting compression garment, which should be worn for 24 hours a day, including overnight, for four to six weeks after surgery. Your garment will have vents so that it may be worn even when using the restroom. The garment may be washed on the gentle cycle and air-dried as needed. While this is being done, stay off your feet and minimize activity.

You may be discharged home with drains—proper drain care is required. Follow the instructions given to you by your doctor and nurse. The JP (Jackson-Pratt) drain helps drain excess blood and fluid from under the skin at the incision site. This drain will stay in place for approximately one week or until the drainage has slowed down or stopped. Your doctor will decide when it is time to remove it.

After healing occurs, the fluid will change color; it starts out red and gradually turns yellow.

Keep the drain pinned to your clothing/binder to keep it from being pulled out.

Empty the drain at least twice a day and keep track of how much fluid has been dumped out of each drain.

Gently clean around each drain with mild soap and water, rinse well, and then keep the area dry.

Call your doctor if there is greater than 400 ccs/mls of drainage in a 24-hour period.

No tub soaking while drains or sutures are present.

It is not uncommon for your genitals, legs, and feet to become swollen and/or bruised after surgery. If this seems excessive, contact your physician.

Avoid sex for two weeks after surgery, and then have sex very carefully for the next two weeks.

Driving is permitted starting one to two weeks after surgery, if you feel well and are not taking prescription pain medication or sedatives.

If you are employed, expect to take at least seven to 10 days off work.

Do not use a hot tub or sauna for four weeks after surgery. You may enter a swimming pool after two weeks, but no swimming for four to six weeks.

Massage to Decrease Swelling in the Legs

Massage treatment to decrease swelling in the legs is appropriate after liposuction of the thigh, liposuction of the knee or lower leg, calf augmentation, thigh lift, or any surgery performed on the lower extremity. See Photo 1 to guide you when performing the pre-treatment massage techniques. This shows the directions in which you guide the fluid to the lymph nodes.

Step 1. Pre-Treatment Massage

The following four steps will be performed at the start of every treatment session, no matter what area of the body you are working on.

Perform in this order: collarbone, side of neck, back of neck, and deep breathing, all as described in Chapter 10 and below.

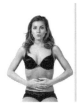 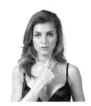 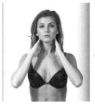 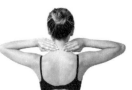

Photo 1A-D: Pre-treatment Massage

A. Deep breathing

Deep breathing is done by contracting the diaphragm.

Begin by placing both hands flat on your belly, over your diaphragm.

Inhale slowly—breathe deeply through your nose, allowing your stomach to expand into your hand.

As air enters your lungs, your abdomen—not your chest wall—should expand outwards.

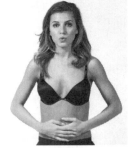

Breathe out slowly through pursed lips, allowing your stomach to flatten.

Repeat five times with a short rest between each breath to avoid dizziness.

Photo 2: Deep breathing

B. Collarbone (clavicle)

Place the bottom of your second (index) and third (middle) fingers on either side of your neck just above your collarbone.

Stroke down towards your collarbone and inward toward your neck. Stretch

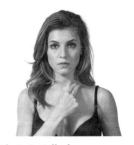

Photo 3: Collarbone massage

the skin just as far as it naturally goes. This stroke would look like two "J" strokes facing one another.

This technique can be applied on both sides at the same time or on one side at a time.

If doing both sides at the same time, you may find it more comfortable to cross your arms while you do this stroke.

Repeat 15 times.

C. Side of neck

Place the bottom of your hands on either side of your neck just under your ears and gently stretch the skin down towards your collarbone and release.

Keep a slow and rhythmic pace.

Repeat this stroke 10 to 15 times.

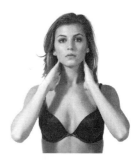

Photo 4: Massaging the side of the neck

D. Back of neck

Place the bottom of your hands on the back of your neck just below your hairline on either side of your spine.

Stretch the skin towards the spine and then down toward base of neck and release.

Repeat 10 to 15 times.

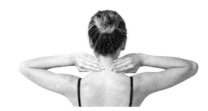

Photo 5: Massaging the back of the neck

Step 2. Groin Lymph Nodes

Lie on your back. Bend your leg slightly and then place your hand on the angle that forms between your leg and pelvis.

Place your fingertips on this crease. Your hand is placed just below the hipbone, but closer to your private area.

Make circles for two to three minutes.

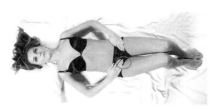

Photo 6: Massaging the groin lymph nodes

Step 3. Outer Hip Lymph Nodes

Lie on your back. Bend your leg slightly and then place your hand on the bony area on the outer hip. Make circles for two to three minutes, directing the pressure toward your belly.

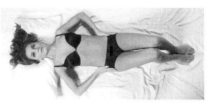

Photo 7: Massaging the outer hip lymph nodes

Step 4. Outside of Upper Thigh

With a flat hand, lightly drag your hand on the outside of your thigh and hip, toward your hip.

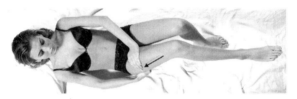

Photo 8: Massaging the outside of the upper thigh

Step 5. Inside of Thigh Outwards

Starting on the inside of your upper thigh, make stationary circles and massage towards the outside of your thigh.

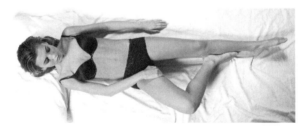

Photo 9: Massaging inside of upper thigh

Step 6. Above Knee

Make stationary circles just above your knee, starting on the inside and moving towards the outside of your thigh.

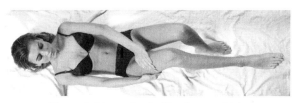

Photo 10: Massaging inside of upper thigh

Step 7. Lower Outer Thigh

Make stationary circles with your hand flat against the outside of your thigh.

Start just above the knee and stroke upward towards the hip.

Pressure is directed from the knee towards the hip.

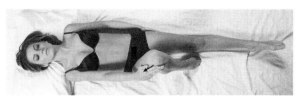

Photo 11: Massaging the lower outer thigh

Step 8. Back of Knee

Make stationary circles with the flats of your hands, behind your knee.

Pressure is directed gently upwards toward the thigh.

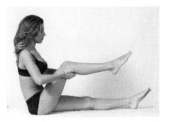

Photo 12: Massaging the back of your knee

Step 9. Outside and Inside of Knee

Make stationary circles with the flats of your fingers, gently stroking the inside and outside of your knee.

Pressure is directed towards the thigh.

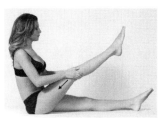

Photo 13: Massaging the inside and outside of your knee

Step 10. Lower Leg

Make stationary circles with the flat of your hand on the inner and outer surface of your lower leg (your calf).

Direct the strokes upwards towards your knee.

Massage the entire area from your ankle to your knee.

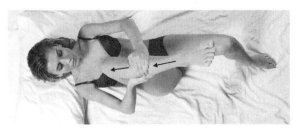

Photo 14: Massaging the lower leg

Step 11. Top of the Foot

Make stationary circles on the top of the foot.

Direct the strokes toward the ankle.

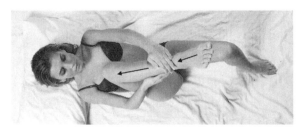

Photo 15: Massaging the top of the foot

Step 12. Go Back Up Entire Leg

Repeat strokes going from ankle back up the entire leg to the groin.

Section Five
Experiences

Chapter 19
My Personal Experience

When I made the decision to have plastic surgery, I figured I would be in for a rough adventure. I decided to keep track of my entire experience. Here are the journal entries and pictures I kept throughout my journey. I had laser body sculpting (liposuction) of my abdomen, back, and upper arm.

My Decision

*This shouldn't be so hard. I work out every day...well, almost every day. I am being crazy about my diet and exercise. This is nuts. Why can't I lose these love handles? I guess it's my lot in life. My dad has it, my grandmother had it...it's inevitable I will too. There must be an alternative...*I decide to consult a plastic surgeon.

Meet with the Surgeon

I meet with the doctor. He answers all my questions and concerns. He gives me options...best option is laser-assisted liposuction. Surgery scheduled.

Prepare Myself Before Surgery

Today I need to go shopping. I've got to get my ice ready, food prepared, garment, and medications I need. I think it would be hard to get this stuff together after surgery.

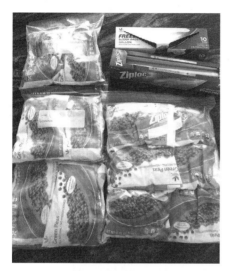

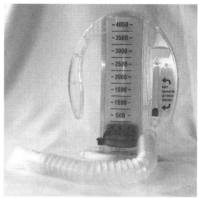

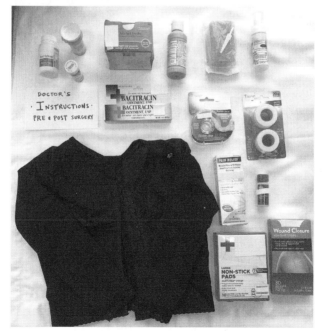

Photo 1A-C: Things I bought to prepare before surgery

I wonder how I am going to look after surgery compared to before. I better take some pictures before.

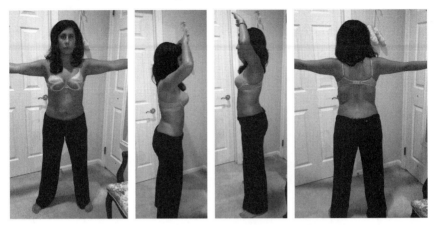

Photo 2A-D: "Before" pictures taken the night before surgery

Surgery Day

Tuesday. Day of surgery...no food before surgery. I'm not even hungry. I am too nervous. Get my things together...My brother George escorts me to the surgery center. Arrive...fill out paperwork in the waiting room.

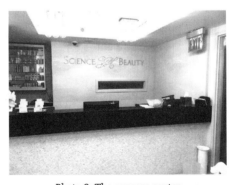

Photo 3: The surgery center

Taken into pre-op holding area. Change into gown, hat, and booties. I sit there and wait for the next step. Met with anesthesiologist. Discussed with him the fact that I am easily affected by anesthesia and that I often vomit after waking up from surgery.

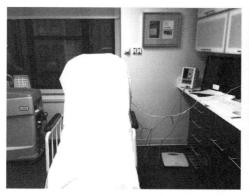

Photo 4: The Pre-op room

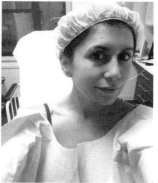

Photo 5: Me in hat and
gown waiting for the
anesthesiologist and doctor

Doctor marks me for surgery—flashback memory of rushing a sorority and hearing rumors that the "sisters" would circle your fat in public as a hazing stunt—it never happened. Fast forward years later—here I am getting my fat circled in public—sweet.

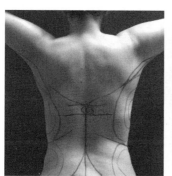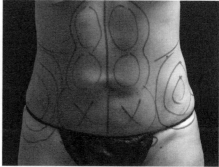

Photo 6A-B: The doctor circles my "problem areas"

Taken into OR...talking to doctor...he makes me feel very calm...nurses are very sweet and one holds my hand...IV started...drift off to sleep.

Nurse wakes me up...confused for a minute where I am. Felt no pain, but had a hard time catching my breath—garments are tight. Sat up...started coughing and felt something stuck in my chest but nothing coming out. Asked nurse to do chest PT on my back. Coughed out bloody junk. Ah relief. Did not feel much pain.

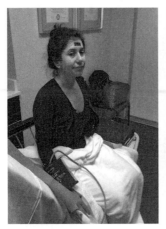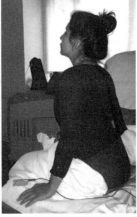

Photo 7A-B: Sitting up for the first time after surgery

Brother took me home. Had to put plastic pads down on seats of car because I was draining so much. Had trouble getting out of the car. Rested when I got home. Walked around house. Drank several glasses of water. Slept.

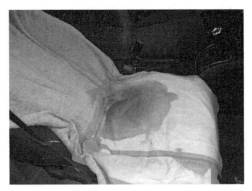

Photo 8: The plastic pad on the car seat with bloody drainage

Day #1 after Surgery

Wednesday. Pain set in—woah! Took some Tylenol. Didn't want heavy pain meds—Vicodin—Tylenol was good enough. So much difficulty moving. Couldn't cook or make my own lunch. Walked around house every couple hours for circulation. Needed "maximum assist" to get out of bed or couch. Swelling in thighs, abdomen, sides, and back. Started drinking eight to 10 glasses of water daily. Did deep breathing and ankle pumps.

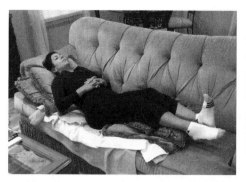
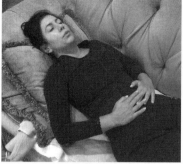

Photo 9A-B: Day 1 after surgery resting, doing my ankle pumps and deep breathing

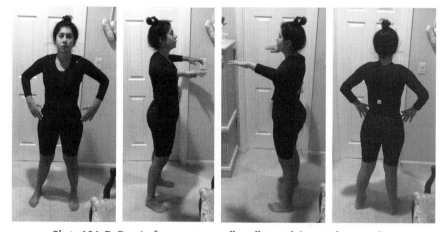

Photo 10A-D: Day 1 after surgery, swollen all over, doing gentle arm raises

Day #2 after Surgery

Thursday. Very swollen! Needed "moderate assist" to get out of bed. Took garment off but my blood pressure dropped and I almost passed out. Good thing my family was there to help me! Applied arnica gel. Continued drinking water. Had one small coffee. Needed a lot of help to change my bandages. Started gentle arm raises.

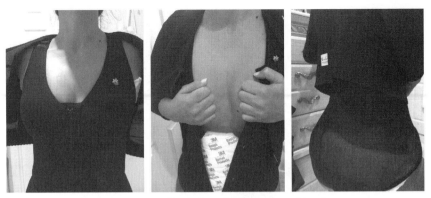

Photo 11A-C: Needing help to change pads and bandages

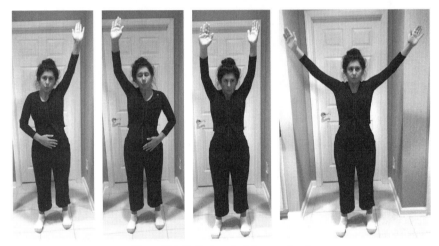

Photo 12A-D: Doing stretches on day 2

Day #3 after Surgery

Friday. Still needed help from my family to get out of bed. Showered with my mom checking in on me to make sure I didn't faint, and I didn't—win. Started peeing a good amount. Started walking more around the house. Walked one to two blocks. Continued water. Took garment off and had a lot of pooled swelling (seroma) in my lower stomach. Started lymphatic massage on myself and the swelling in my stomach went down a lot.

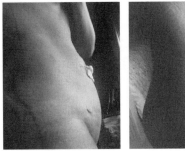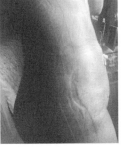

Photo 13A-B: Swelling pooled in my stomach before and then after massage

Day #4 after Surgery

Saturday. Easier moving around. Still need a little bit of help to get out of bed. Massage. Still some swelling in back and sides. Put on abdominal binder over garment to target swelling in this area. Getting more sensation back everywhere. Increased walking.

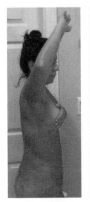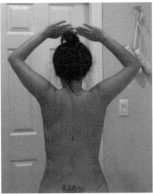

Photo 14A-B: Swelling and bruising is improving but still in back and sides

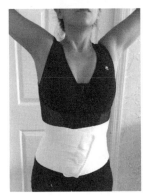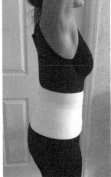

Photo 15A-B: Wearing abdominal binder over my garment

Day #5 after Surgery

Sunday. Able to get out of bed and move around independently. Very itchy all over—had to take a Benadryl. Incisions and stitches itch. Massage. Peeing more. My endurance is decreased from my baseline. Increased walking. When I walk around without the garment—only before and after shower—it feels like there is a five-to-eight-pound phantom weight belt around me.

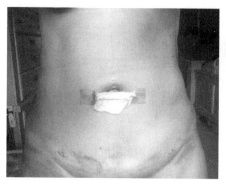 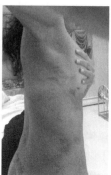

Photo 16A-B: Swelling and bruising in stomach and sides improving

Day #6 after Surgery

Monday. Same. Itchy. I see big improvements today. More range of motion exercises, stretching to end of range. Lower back and lower abdomen are numb. Increased walking distance.

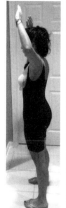 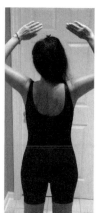 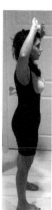 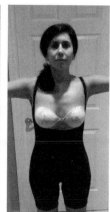 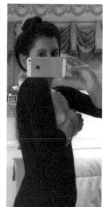

Photo 17A-D: Doing stretches on day 6

Day #7 after Surgery

Tuesday. Started to feel knotty areas where connective tissue was beginning to re-adhere. Very tight all over! Had difficulty lifting arms. Small lumpy nodules appeared under the skin on my abdomen, sides, and underarms. I massaged them until they were flat. Had to massage those areas to prevent a lumpy abdomen. Increased walking. Preparing to return to work.

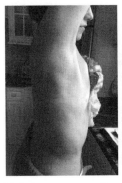 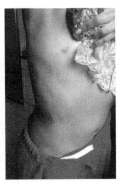

Photo 18A-B: Lumps start to form and the skin is getting very tight

Day #8 after Surgery

Wednesday. Today is the one-week postoperative visit with my doctor. Stitches removed. Returned to work for half a day. Walked 10 city blocks and five avenues twice.

Day #9 after Surgery

Thursday: Lost more water weight, most likely due to the increase in walking combined with the 10 glasses of water daily.

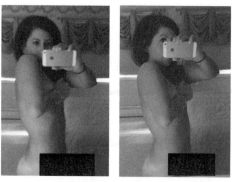

Photo 20A-B: Day 9 photos with no bruising and less swelling

Day #10 after Surgery

Friday. Tightness around my body really set in. Did 30 minutes of stretching—lots of stretching. Felt better after stretching.

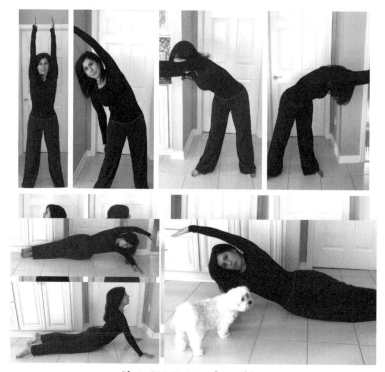

Photo 21A-D: Lots of stretching

Day #11 after Surgery

Saturday. Continued lots of stretching and massage.

Day #12 after Surgery

Sunday. Lots of walking, stretching, and massage. Go to my aunt's house. She makes a dinner of chicken in a marsala sauce, rice pilaf with bullion, and salad. Realized it was a very salty meal. I start to feel puffy soon after I am done eating. My garment starts to feel tight around my body. I start to feel uncomfortable.

Day #13 after Surgery

Monday. Woke up so swollen, all over, due to salty dinner. Ate low-salt again. Thinking the salty dinner was not worth the effects, even two weeks out of surgery. Drank water. Need to get the salt and swelling out of my body. Start running today. Put on abdominal binder in addition to garment. After my run I am changing in the bathroom and I hear something and feel a weird sensation. All of a sudden I notice clear, yellow fluid shooting out of my incision sites. I had no idea what was happening. Then I realized I "sprung a leak." The crazy amounts of swelling, from yesterday, were coming out of the path of least resistance—the incisions. I thought the incisions were totally closed up—but to my surprise they kept leaking.

Day #14 after Surgery

Tuesday. Lost four pounds since yesterday—all the fluid that poured out of the incisions. I am still puffy compared to a couple days ago, but not bad. I started wearing a more intense abdominal binder. Started jogging today.

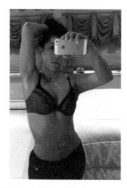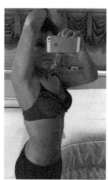

Photo 22A-B: Still puffy from salty dinner–but coming back from it

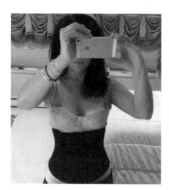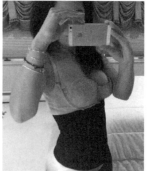

Photo 23A-B: Start wearing tighter abdominal binder

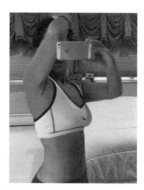

Photo 24: Started jogging today

Day #15 after Surgery

Thursday. Got a haircut. Feel and look so much thinner. Went out. Got overwhelming feedback about how thin and skinny I look compared to normal. One guy friend said, "It's unbelievable how different you look."

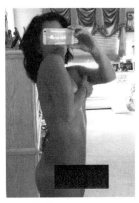

Photo 25: Day 15 photo

Day #30 after Surgery

One month post-op. I look different. Still have swelling—lower abdomen puffy but less swelling in other places after doing lymphatic massage. Still in all garments. Still wearing abdominal binder over garments.

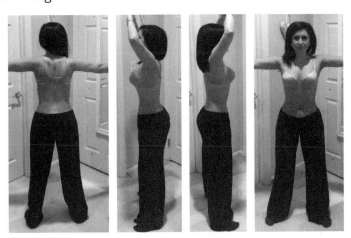

Photo 26A-D: Day 30 After photos

And the progress continues...

Chapter 20
Patient Experiences

This chapter contains two parts:

Part One: *Examples from my notes about two different patients*

Part Two: *Testimonials from my patients over the years*

Part One: My Case Notes

The following are examples of notes I have kept on patients over the years.

I begin by showing you the template I use to document my patients' recovery. Within this template I record the patient's name, age, and important information.

I then take a thorough medical history. This is important because the medical history will let me know if there is any reason I cannot treat the patient. For example, if a patient recently has had active cancer, I cannot perform massage on them because it puts them at risk for spreading the cancer through the lymphatic system. Other medical conditions are also important for me to know.

I also need to know the medications the patient is taking. This gives me valuable information on side effects they may be experiencing.

I then make sure to document the exact surgery performed, which body areas had surgery and the date of the surgery, so I know how far along they are in the recovery process.

I then take note of the patient's subjective complaints. This means I record what the patient says and how they feel. This is a typical practice of all physical therapists.

I then take objective data. I note areas of swelling and take exact measurements with a tape measure. I also note limitations in function, i.e. if they cannot get out of bed, stand, or walk well; limitations in range of motion, i.e. if they cannot lift their arm all the way; and any areas of bruising. After I have taken the objective data, I make a list of their problems. These problems will show me, the physical therapist, exactly what I have to treat.

I then make a plan for the treatment of these problems—my treatment plan for that patient.

At each follow-up visit I note how the patient is progressing—specifically if and how their problems are getting better.

Don't worry if you find this a little confusing—it took me years of schooling to figure out how to do this.

Case Notes about Two Real Patients

Patient One: Sam

Initial Evaluation date: *May 21, 2013 notes*

Sam is a 51-year-old male who presents on post-op day 11 after liposuction of the medial thighs and flanks. After performing Sam's initial evaluation, I generated a list of the problems assessed. I then provided a solution for each problem listed.

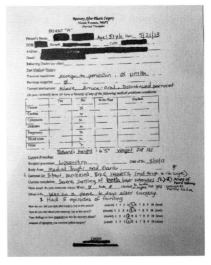

Problem #1: Patient purchased bike shorts and is wearing them instead of a medical compression garment.

Photo 1: Initial evaluation of Sam

Solution to #1: I educated Sam in this session on the detrimental effects of wearing the wrong compression. I informed him that the bike shorts caused uneven pressure, trapping swelling in his leg, which now developed into non-pitting edema. I directed Sam to a professional medical supply company in his area (NYC) where he could be fitted for the proper garment.

Problem #2: Sam's diet consists of no water. He is consuming alcohol every night, salt, and ice teas as his primary means of hydration.

Solution to #2: Educated Sam on the proper diet of water, water with lemon, low salt, restricting his alcohol intake (ideally no alcohol consumption). His current diet is contributing to the severe fluid retention he is experiencing. The iced tea is dehydrating his body, which also contributes to retention of fluid.

Problem #3: Severe swelling of the lower extremities with hardening of the tissue where it has accumulated. The left leg was larger than the right leg.

Problem #4: Patient was on a plane six days after surgery.

Problem #5: Patient had five episodes of fainting.

Solution to Problems #3, #4, and #5: Severe swelling of the lower extremities is a concern in itself; but swelling that is greater in one leg than the other could indicate a potential blood clot.

Assessment

The patient is a 51-year-old male who presents s/p liposuction of both legs. The patient presents with severe swelling, pain, redness in the lower extremities, with the left leg presenting larger. The patient was on a plane for greater than three hours, six days after surgery. He has had five episodes of fainting. These are red flags and therefore I did not perform any manual therapy during this session and referred the patient immediately back to his surgeon. I personally called the surgeon during the session to relay the findings. The doctor asked that the patient immediately return to his office for an examination.

Follow up: *The doctor took the necessary steps to treat a DVT in the patient's leg and placed the patient on a blood thinner. After a few days, the doctor cleared the patient of any medical issues or concerns and okayed the patient to resume treatment and lymphatic massage. Fainting was determined by the doctor to be due to the Percocet. The doctor okayed sessions to resume on May 24, 2013.*

May 24, 2013 Notes from Treatment Session

Subjective

> *"I am better now. I am glad you caught
> the blood clot in my leg."*

Objective

May 24, 2013— *Measurements taken BEFORE treatment*	**May 24, 2013—** *Measurements taken AFTER treatment*

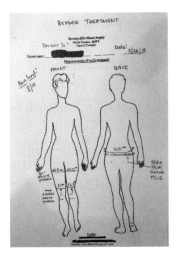

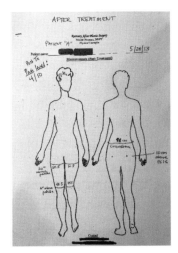

Photo 2: Measurements taken BEFORE treatment	*Photo 3: Measurements taken AFTER treatment*

Difference of circumferential girth measurements after treatment as compared to before treatment in centimeters (cm)

Right thigh

6 cm above patella .... 2.5 cm smaller

20 cm above patella .... 2.0 cm smaller

Left thigh

6 cm above patella .... 3.8 cm smaller

20 cm above patella .... 2.2 cm smaller

Waist

10 cm above PSIS.. 7.0 cm smaller

Response to Treatment

Sam tolerated the session well with no adverse response. His pain level reduced from an 8/10 to a 4/10 in one session. He verbalized a feeling of increased range of motion and increased ease with mobility—getting off the couch and walking.

Assessment

The patient is a 51-year-old male who presents status post-liposuction of the medial thighs and flanks, on post-op Day 14. The patient presents with edema in the lower extremities (left greater than right), hardening of the tissue, decreased range of motion, decreased flexibility, and increased pain which are affecting his ability to transfer in and out of bed, ambulate, transfer on and off the toilet, take on and off his clothing, and perform his ADLs. Factors contributing to these impairments include improper garment, improper diet, and recent trip on a plane for greater than three hours. This patient would benefit from skilled PT intervention combined with education to achieve his goals of improved appearance, improved flexibility, improved gait, and ease with ADLs.

Plan of Care

The patient will require multiple treatments (three times a week) following the first treatment session. Treatment will include: lymphatic massage performed by the therapist, and therapist instructed the patient in self-lymphatic massage. Also included in treatment will be decongestive exercises to perform two to three times a day. Sam obtained the correct compression garment after the initial assessment and is educated on a wearing schedule and proper skin care. His treatment will also include reviewing education on diet, increasing water intake, and decreasing sodium, alcohol, and iced tea consumption.

Patient Two: Christina

Initial Evaluation: *August 5, 2013 notes*

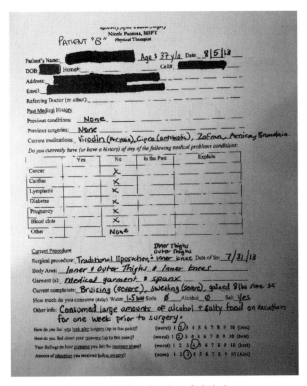

Photo 4: Initial evaluation of Christina

Subjective

"My legs are massive and so black and bruised! I went on vacation before surgery, had cocktails and relaxed. Why did this happen to me?"

Objective

August 5, 2013—
*Measurements taken
BEFORE treatment*

August 5, 2013—
*Measurements taken
AFTER treatment*

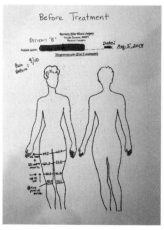

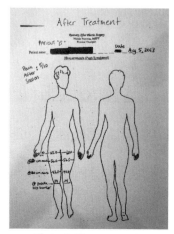

Photo 5: Measurements
taken BEFORE treatment

Photo 6: Measurements
taken AFTER treatment

Difference of circumferential girth measurements after treatment as compared to before treatment in centimeters (cm)

Right leg

Superior border of patella .... 1.5 cm smaller

10 cm above patella .... 7.0 cm smaller

20 cm above patella .... 4.0 cm smaller

30 cm above the patella................................... 1.5 cm smaller

Left leg

Superior border of patella .... 0.5 cm smaller

10 cm above patella .... 1.5 cm smaller

20 cm above patella .... 1.5 cm smaller

30 cm above patella .... 0 cm (no change)

Intervention

Christina is a 37-year-old female who presents on post-op day five after liposuction of the medial and lateral thighs and inner knees. After performing Christina's initial evaluation, I generated a list of the problems assessed. I then provided a solution for each problem listed.

Problem #1: Christina consumed large amounts of alcohol prior to surgery resulting in severe ecchymosis (bruising) on the anterior, posterior, lateral, and medial thighs.

Solution to #1: I educated Christina in this session on the detrimental effects of consuming alcohol prior to surgery. I informed educated her on the benefits of oral and topical Arnica Montana. I used Arnica during the session.

Problem #2: Christina has severe postoperative swelling.

Solution to #2: Educated Christina on the proper diet of water, water with lemon, low salt, restricting all alcohol consumption. I performed lymphatic drainage massage, educated her on a garment wearing schedule, and initiated basic decongestive exercises. She was also educated on the benefits of Bromelain and pineapple as a natural supplement to reduce swelling.

Christina tolerated the session well with sensitivity to lymphatic massage and palpation of lymph nodes, which became tolerable after several minutes. Her pain level reduced from a 9/10 to a 5/10 in one session. At the end of the session she expressed feeling overjoyed because she could sit on the toilet and get off the toilet without her husband helping her.

Assessment

The patient is a 37-year-old female who presents on post-op day five after liposuction of the medial and lateral thighs and inner knees. The patient presents with severe swelling and ecchymosis in the lower extremities decreased range of motion, decreased flexibility, and increased pain which are affecting her ability to transfer on and off the toilet, ambulate, get in and out of bed, don/doff her clothing, and perform her ADLs. Factors contributing to these impairments include: improper consumption of alcohol and salty food prior to surgery, and improper diet currently. This patient would benefit from skilled PT intervention combined with education to achieve her goals of improved appearance, improved flexibility, improved gait, and ease with ADLs.

Plan of Care

The patient will require daily treatments following the first treatment session. Treatment will include lymphatic massage performed by the therapist and instruct the patient in self-lymphatic massage every other day, alternating with a regimen of decongestive exercises. Christina's treatment will also include reviewing education on diet, increasing water intake, and decreasing sodium and alcohol consumption.

August 6, 2013 Notes from Treatment Session

Subjective

> *"I lost four pounds since yesterday!"*

Objective

Difference of circumferential girth measurements after treatment as compared to before treatment in centimeters (cm)

Right leg

Superior border of patella .... 0 cm (no change)

10 cm above patella .... 0.5 cm smaller

20 inches above patella .... 1.5 cm smaller

30 cm above patella .... 1.0 cm smaller

Left leg

Superior border of patella ....0 cm (no change)

10 cm above patella .... 1.0 cm smaller

20 cm above patella .... 2.5 cm smaller

30 cm above patella .... 2.0 cm smaller

Interventions

Instruction in self-lymphatic drainage massage, performed decongestive exercises of legs and abdomen, applied topical Arnica gel, and reviewed all education.

Response

Christina tolerated the session very well with no sensitivity to self-lymphatic massage and decongestive exercise. Her pain level was a 4/10 today and she was extremely excited that she had lost four pounds of fluid. She expressed a feeling of increased flexibility and ease of movement.

Impression

The patient is a 37-year-old female who presents on post-op day five after liposuction of the medial and lateral thighs and inner knees. Since yesterday the patient has lost four pounds of fluid, shown a decrease in girth and increased flexibility, range of motion, resulting in improved gait pattern, ability to transfer in an out of bed, improved ability to get on and off the toilet, and she is now able to don and doff her clothes independently. She continues to benefit from physical therapy intervention.

Plan of Care

The patient continues to benefit from daily treatments that will include lymphatic massage performed by the therapist and instruct the patient in self-lymphatic massage every other day, alternating with a regimen of decongestive exercises. Christina's treatment will also include reviewing education on diet, increasing water intake, and decreasing sodium and alcohol consumption.

August 12, 2013 Notes from Re-Evaluation Session

Subjective

"I feel like myself again and finally see the results of the surgery. I have no pain and I can walk like I did before the surgery."

Objective

Difference in girth measurements at initial evaluation (8/05/13) compared to today (8/12/13) in centimeters (cm)

Right leg	8/5	8/12	Difference
Superior border of patella	35.5	34.0	1.5 cm smaller
10 cm above patella	50.5	42.0	8.5 cm smaller
20 cm above patella	60.0	50.5	9.5 cm smaller
30 cm above patella	64.5	55.0	9.5 cm smaller

Left leg	8/5	8/12	Difference
Superior border of patella	34.5	34.0	0.5 cm smaller
10 cm above patella	45.5	40.5	0.5 cm smaller
20 cm above patella	58.0	49.5	0.5 cm smaller
30 cm above patella	56.0	60.0	4.0 cm smaller

Assessment

The patient is a 37-year-old female who presents Post-op Day #12 after liposuction of the medial and lateral thighs and inner knees. Since the initial evaluation the patient has shown marked reduction in postoperative swelling and girth measurements. She has demonstrated the ability to perform all functional mobility independently, has no pain, and has significantly less bruising. She is now independent with all self-massage, exercises, and diet.

Plan of Care

Review home program and discontinue physical therapy services at this time.

Part Two: Patient Testimonials

Here are some words and feedback from patients I have treated.

I had a tummy tuck done and I thought that it was going to be a quick and painless process with a speedy recovery. I even had a trip to Puerto Rico planned for the week after surgery. The days after surgery were awful! I did not realize that I would be in so much pain. I was so bloated and I could hardly move. I called my surgeon and he told me to give Nicole a call. In our first session I was extremely sensitive and I told her that my pain was at an eight out of 10. After our first session I felt a lot better, and by the next day my pain was at a four out of 10, and I looked so much better. Nicole taught me the reality of my recovery and I quickly realized that Puerto Rico was not an option. We worked together for a few more sessions and my results have been amazing! My surgeon was phenomenal, but Nicole was also an amazing addition to my experience.

—Sarah

I learned about Nicole from a friend of mine who had used her, and I made sure to book my appointments before I even went in for surgery. In our first phone conversation, Nicole talked me through the process and told me what to expect before, during, and after my facelift. Working with her was the best decision I ever made and my surgeon has been so happy with my recovery.

—Beverly

I didn't think of laser liposuction as a real surgery because I purchased it on Groupon® and research on the internet says you can have it done on your lunch break. But after having had one, I am here to tell you that it is! I thought I would have a flat stomach a few days after surgery, but that was not the case. I was swollen and lumpy and I cried for two days straight. Nicole made my recovery so much easier and I know that I would not look this good without her help.

—Bree

I'm back in Kuwait and my thighs feel better and started to shrink also. Thanks to you my dear. I'm doing self-massage every other day and expecting an English lady to come to see me for lymphatic drainage massage next week. I just hope she's good though I know she won't be as good as you. I miss your magic touch. Thank you for the exercises.

—Sahar

I always wanted to get breast implants, but I was so fearful of what they would look like; I didn't want them to look fake or feel hard. After my surgery, Nicole worked with me and I am so happy that I called her because I would not have been able to do this on my own. She is such a professional, and because of her help, I am now one of the 'before and after' photos on my doctor's website.

—Chrissy

I had a body lift done and it felt like I was hit by a bus and I couldn't move. Nicole worked with me for a number of weeks and it was the best call I ever made. She is so good at what she does and I am so happy with my results. If I ever have another procedure done, there is no doubt I will be calling Nicole.

—Laura

I was given a one-page sheet explaining my recovery—thank God I found Nicole to give me better guidance.

—Maya

I had an emergency appendectomy done and my surgeon decided to cut me instead of doing it laparoscopically. After a week of recovery, I got the staples out and I noticed that my incision sight was lumpy and hard. Nicole taught me how to massage the incision sight, and at my second check up with my surgeon, he was amazed at how I was healing. Thanks to Nicole, you can hardly see my scar.

—Greg

In one of our sessions Nicole told me that she was writing a book on these techniques and my first thought was, Wow, this is going to help so many people who have no idea what to expect after plastic surgery, and my second thought was, Well, there goes my secret weapon. Seriously, this is great, Nicole is a miracle worker.

—Sophie

I told all of my friends about my surgery because I am thrilled with my decision. Maybe talking about it will inspire one of them.

—Holly

I was telling people about my surgeries, but now I have decided not to because I feel like they are judging me. After talking to Nicole she made me realize that it is okay if I don't want to share this decision with friends. She explained it is a personal choice that is no one's business but my own.

—Jenna

The media makes plastic surgery seem so glamorous and easy—they lied.

—Tricia

Nicole is so real and down to earth and she was very open about sharing her personal experiences with plastic surgery.

—Alana

I didn't want to tell anyone about the procedure that I had done, but when my best friend confided in me about her plans for a facelift, I felt like I had to tell her about Nicole.

—Mary

Last summer I got an arm lift. I was so excited to have the surgery because I've always been uncomfortable with my flabby arms. My goal for having the surgery was to finally be able to go sleeveless! After the surgery I was extremely distraught. My hands got extremely swollen and although I knew there might be scarring, I didn't realize how apparent it would be. I was devastated that the surgery I had wanted all my life was the worst thing I did. Nicole was completely amazing in helping me post-surgery. Not only did she help to reduce the swelling in my hands, she also helped me to eliminate the scarring! She knew exactly what to say and do to make me feel comfortable and let me see that I would be happy with my decision to have surgery; I just had to be patient with the recovery. Now I am looking forward to this summer filled with a new wardrobe of sleeveless outfits—all without my friends and family knowing a thing!

—Jen

Nicole—I just wanted to let you know I urinated a ton last night and this morning. The swollen part above my scar is almost completely flat! I know it might swell a little after being on my feet a lot today, but I just finally feel like I am actually actively recovering and not just trying to get by. Thank you so much!!!

—Melissa

Nicole and her smile, aliveness, pleasure in her work, flexibility, good humor, and her insistence. Nicole never gave up; she insisted I do things and I stuck with her and practiced in between sessions with her, sometimes feeling like I hated her despite her beautiful face and personality. I was in pain and I felt hopeless and in a bad humor, and she was telling me to do things that were hard. Nicole worked with me and my moods tirelessly; I worked very hard; and other than how much I loved Nicole, I hated the work and the pain. Results: I am back to myself and better than before, am active, go to the gym, do exercises and stretches to keep myself in shape, and have my professional and personal life back. Nicole, I will always be grateful to you; I'm not just saying this for your book.

—**Michael**